NUREG/CP-0177
PNNL-13654

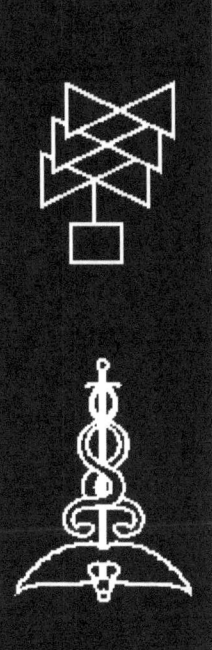

Proceedings of the Environmental Software Systems Compatibility and Linkage Workshop

Hosted by
The U.S Nuclear Regulatory Commission
NRC Professional Development Center
Rockville, Maryland
March 7–9, 2000

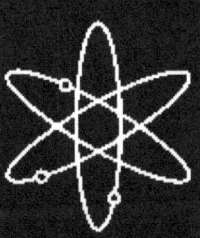

Pacific Northwest National Laboratory

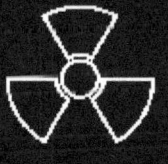

U.S. Nuclear Regulatory Commission
Office of Nuclear Regulatory Research
Washington, DC 20555-0001

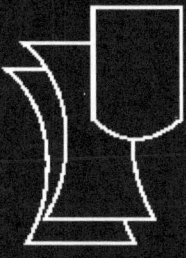

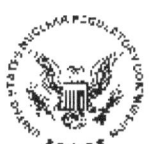

NUREG/CP-0177
PNNL-13654

Proceedings of the Environmental Software Systems Compatibility and Linkage Workshop

Hosted by
The U.S. Nuclear Regulatory Commission
NRC Professional Development Center
Rockville, Maryland
March 7–9, 2000

Manuscript Completed: September 2001
Date Published: May 2002

Edited by
Gene Whelan, PNNL

Thomas J. Nicholson, NRC

Pacific Northwest National Laboratory
Richland, WA 99352

Prepared for
Division of Systems Analysis and Regulatory Effectiveness
Office of Nuclear Regulatory Research
U.S. Nuclear Regulatory Commission
        Washington, DC 20555-0001

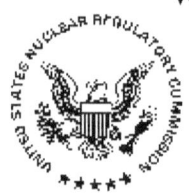

MAY 2002

PROCEEDINGS OF THE ENVIRONMENTAL SOFTWARE
SYSTEMS COMPATIBILITY AND LINKAGE WORKSHOP
MARCH 7–9, 2000

NUREG/CP-0177

ABSTRACT

The NRC hosted a Federal interagency workshop on multimedia environmental software systems and data systems. The "Environmental Software Systems Compatibility and Linkage Workshop" was held at NRC 's Professional Development Center in Rockville, MD, on March 7-9, 2000. The environmental software systems that were discussed are used to evaluate contaminant release, transport and health effects through various media (hence multimedia refers to air, ground, and surface water) and environmental pathways to the public. A major motivation for the workshop was the desire of the participating Federal agencies to realize efficiencies and cost savings by utilizing existing models, systems, and databases developed in their programs, rather than developing totally new systems. Workshop participants for this inaugural gathering included Federal agencies, their cooperators and contractors (e.g., U.S. Army Corps of Engineers, EPA's national exposure research laboratories, Offices of Research and Development, Radiation and Indoor Air, Solid Waste and Water, DOE, Pacific Northwest National Laboratory, Argonne National Laboratory, Golder Associates Inc., State of New Jersey and New Jersey Institute of Technology). The workshop objective was to facilitate communication between software products by focusing on standard attributes, protocols and specifications for linking environmental and risk models to databases and modeling systems. The workshop included presentations and demonstrations of current software systems (e.g., RESRAD, MEPAS, FRAMES, SEDSS, DandD, HWIR, LMS, WMS, etc.) used in site decommissioning assessments. The workshop attendees (1) reviewed detailed suggestions from system developers and users on attributes for linking the existing models, systems, Web-based, and GIS databases; and (2) discussed alternative software designs to ensure compatibility and linkage for future models, systems, and datasets. During an evening breakout session, the Federal agency representatives discussed the development of a Memorandum of Understanding (MOU) for cooperating and coordinating research. Following the workshop, the MOU was developed and signed by NRC, EPA, DOE, U.S. Army Corps of Engineers, U.S. Geological Survey, and USDA/Agricultural Research Service, and is now being implemented.

Contents

Appendices

Figures

Tables

Executive Summary

Prepared by D. Brown and K.J. Castleton

This report describes the state of environmental modeling within the government sector as understood by the attendees of the March 7–10, 2000, meeting, also referred to as the *March 2000* workshop. It is important to note that these systems are multiple-environmental-media modeling systems, not single-media modeling systems. These systems models include representations of various media (e.g., air, ground, and surface water). A concise description of each system is given in this document.

Four Federal and one State government agencies and their collaborative groups attended the meeting. The meeting was hosted by the U.S. Nuclear Regulatory Commission (NRC) at its Professional Development Center in Rockville, Maryland on March 7-9, 2000. The participating organizations were:

- US Nuclear Regulatory Commission
  - Office of Nuclear Regulatory Research
  - Office of Nuclear Materials Safety and Safeguards
- US Department of Energy
  - Office of Environmental Management
    - Pacific Northwest National Laboratory
    - Oak Ridge National Laboratory
    - Argonne National Laboratory
- US Environmental Protection Agency
  - Office of Radiation and Indoor Air
  - Office of Research and Development at Athens
  - Office of Solid Waste
  - Office of Water
- US Department of Defense, Army Corps of Engineers, Engineer Research and Development Center - Waterways Experiment Station
- New Jersey Institute of Technology
- New Jersey Department of Environmental Protection
- Golder Associates, Inc.
- Sandford Cohen & Associates

The objective of each group for environmental modeling is given in this report. This set of groups was not seen as complete; it was the network of individuals known to the meeting organizers at the time. Every attempt was made to make the list as complete as possible. In the months following this meeting, the organizers have contacted additional groups that are interested in being involved with the design process.

The activities of the meeting were:

1. Different environmental model development groups presented the current state of their systems.

2. Round table discussions about different attributes of the systems were conducted.

The products of the meeting were:

1. A list of attributes (requirements) that a mutually acceptable and inclusive modeling system addressing needs of the whole group would need to have (See Table 5.1).

2. This report, which describes the current state of these systems and contains the attributes list.

Since the meeting, the list of attributes has been used to make development decisions by groups involved in the original meeting. In a very real sense, this consensus list of attributes has already moved the groups toward a common software framework.

The primary motivation for the meeting itself was to start and encourage a dialog between the participants in the future development of integrated multimedia modeling systems. With resources diminishing in the federal sector, there is a need to develop working relationships between Federal agencies and the commercial sector. A memorandum of understanding is in the process of being signed by six Federal agencies as a result of this meeting and follow-on discussions.

Specific recommendations were identified during the workshop. The recommendations in this report are broken into two categories: 1) organizational and 2) software-system attributes. The software-system attributes are described in detail in Table 5.1, so only the higher level philosophical software recommendations are discussed here.

The list of organizational recommendation includes:

- Multimedia model developers should continue discussions to refine and clarify the attributes. This can be encouraged by having an annual meeting similar to the original meeting, supplemented by more frequent meetings and conference calls between working technical groups.

- The relationship between the Federal agencies involved should be formalized. Some formalization has already been accomplished through development of a memorandum of understanding (MOU) that is now circulating among the participating agencies for a signature.

- No one agency or group should be "in charge" of this collaborative effort toward a unified system. This is an obvious conclusion and a statement of the opinion of the groups involved. It is an obvious conclusion because the group is a collection of equals, but it is important to the group that there is no effort to make one group the managers of the others.

- Make all attempts to make the group involved in this effort complete. If additional multimedia system developers are discovered by the group, every effort should be made to include them. Following this recommendation will allow this group to grow and to develop a more complete and compatible target list of attributes.

Following is the summary of important philosophical software recommendations:

- Many software systems may satisfy the present list of attributes. Likewise, many useful software systems may address only part of the software-system attributes, but only systems that cover all the attributes will be useful to all groups in the meeting.

- Ownership of software systems needs to remain with the originators. This is not just an intellectual property (IP) statement; this statement also implies that the direction that specific software will be taken is controlled by the originator.

- Ownership of project management needs to remain with the users (developers) of the software system. This is to say that project managers still need to be able to control the time frames and application details of their simulation efforts in relation to their governing missions and goals. For example, it would not make sense to allow the development goals of a common system to interrupt the simulation needs of the individual participating Federal agencies.

- The future systems need to honor legacy code. Multimedia software systems cannot require a redevelopment of the models that currently exist. With diminishing resources in the Federal sector, the past investment in these models is a very valuable resource.

This set of recommendations is expected to be refined as the group continues to interact, and a history develops that allows participants to more clearly understand the collective impacts of certain attributes. It is reasonable to assume that the list of attributes might be unattainable with current software technology. That is not presently believed to be the case, but only a history of attempts at implementation will make it clear whether this belief is true.

Acknowledgments

The editors would like to extend their personal gratitude to the following scientists, engineers, and researchers who helped promote and support this workshop:

- Gerard Laniak and David Brown, U.S. Environmental Protection Agency, Office of Research and Development, Ecosystems Research Division
- Ralph Cady and William Ott, and Jack Parrot, U.S. Nuclear Regulatory Commission, Offices of Nuclear Regulatory Research and Nuclear Materials Safety and Safeguards, respectively
- Mark Dortch and Jeff Holland, U.S. Department of Defense, Army Corps of Engineers, Engineer Research and Development Center, Waterways Experiment Station
- Paul Beam, U.S. Department of Energy, Office of Environmental Management
- Joan Adams and Steve Gajewski, Pacific Northwest National Laboratory

Without their unyielding support, multimedia modeling and this workshop would not have been possible. Thanks are also extended to Wayne Cosby, PNNL, and Paula Garrity, NRC, for editing this document. Consolidating the styles of multiple authors into a coherent document is no easy task and greatly appreciated. Pacific Northwest National Laboratory is operated for the U.S. Department of Energy by Battelle under Contract DE-AC06-76RL01830.

Gene Whelan and Tom Nicholson

Abbreviations

3MRA	Multimedia, Multi-pathway, and Multiple receptor Risk Assessment
ANDRA	French radioactive waste management agency
ANL	Argonne National Laboratory
ANSI	American National Standards Institute
API	Applications Programming Interface
ARAMS	Army Risk Assessment Modeling System
ARS	Agricultural Research Service
BCON	Boundary Conditions Processor
BEIS2	Biogenic Emissions Inventory Systems
BEMR	Baseline Environmental Management Report
CAA	Clean Air Act
CADD	Computer Aided Drafting Design
CB	Carbon Bond
CCTM	CMAQ Chemistry Transport Model
CERCLA	Comprehensive Environmental Response, Compensation, and Liability Act
CMAQ	Community Multiscale Air Quality
CMRA	Chemical Migration and Risk Assessment
CORBA	Common Object Request Broker Architecture
COTS	Commercial-off-the-shelf
CRARM	Congressional Commission on Risk Assessment and Risk Management
CSM	Conceptual Site Model
DandD	Decontamination and Decommissioning
DCE	Database Client Editor
DEP	Data Exchange Protocol
DES	DEScription file
DET	Data Extraction Tool
DIAS	Dynamic Information Architecture System
DIC	Data DICtionary File
DoD	U.S. Department of Defense
DOE	U.S. Department of Energy

DOT	Database Owner Tool
ECIP	Emissions-Chemistry Interface Processor
EIS	Environmental Impact Statement
EM	DOE's Office of Environmental Management
EMPRO	Emission Processor
ENRESA	Spanish radioactive waste management agency
EPA	U.S. Environmental Protection Agency
EPA-Athens	EPA's Office of Research and Development at Athens
ERDC	Engineer Research and Development Center (Army Corps of Engineers)
ERED	Environmental Residue-Effects Database
EXPO	Human Exposure Event Model (TRIM)
FAMMOU	Federal Agency Modeling MOU
FaTE	Fate, Transport and Ecological Exposure Model (TRIM)
FRAMES	Framework for Risk Analysis in Multimedia Environmental Systems
FY	Fiscal Year
GENII	GENeration II (computer code)
GID	Global Input Data
GIS	Geographic Information System
GMS	DoD's Groundwater Modeling System
GRF	Global Results File
GUI	Graphical User Interface
HAP	Hazardous Air Pollutant
HEM	Human Exposure Model
HRA-EIS	Hanford Remedial Action Environmental Impact Statement
html	Hypertext Markup Language
http	Hypertext Transfer Protocol
HWIR	Hazardous Waste Identification Rule
IAG	Interagency Agreement
ICON	Initial Conditions Processor
ICRP	International Commission on Radiological Protection
IDA	Inventory Data Analyzer
INER	Taiwanese radioactive waste management agency

INPRO	Input Emission Processor
I/O	Input/Output
IRIS	Integrated Risk Information System
IRRP	Installation Restoration Research Program
ISO	International Standards Organization
JNC	Japan Nuclear Cycle Development Institute
JPROC	Photolysis Rate Processor
LMS	Land Management System
LUPROC	Land-Use Processor
MCEEA	Multimedia Contaminant Environmental Exposure Assessment
MCIP	Meteorology-Chemistry Interface Processor
MEPAS	Multimedia Environmental Pollutant Assessment System
MEPPRO	Models-3 Emission Projections Processor
MEPPS	Models-3 Emission Projection and Processing System
MIMS	Multimedia Integration Modeling System
MOU	Memorandum Of Understanding
MMR	Massachusetts Military Reservation
MRC	Military Relevant Compound
M&S	Modeling and Simulation
MUI	Model-specific User Interface
NAAQS	National Ambient Air Quality StandardsNATANational Air Toxics Assessment
NERL	EPA's National Exposure Research Laboratory
NMSS	NRC's Office of Nuclear Materials Safety and Safeguards
NRC	U.S. Nuclear Regulatory Commission
NRC-RES	NRC's Office of Nuclear Regulatory Research
NRC-NMSS	NRC's Office of Nuclear Materials Safety and Safeguards
OAQPS	EPA's Office of Air Quality Planning and Standards
OGDI	Open Geospatial Database Interchange
ORD	EPA's Office of Research and Development
ORIA	EPA's Office of Radiation and Indoor Air
OGIS	Open Geodata Interoperability Standards
ORNL	Oak Ridge National Laboratory

OS	Operating System
OSW	EPA's Office of Solid Waste
OSWER	Office of Solid Waste and Emergency Response
OUTPRO	Output Processor
OW	EPA's Office of Water
PA	Performance Assessment
PCDF	Primary Communication Data File
PAVE	Package for Analysis and Visualization of Environmental Data
PEIS	Programmatic Environmental Impact Statement
pdf	Probability Distribution Function
PNNL	Pacific Northwest National Laboratory
PROCAN	Process Analysis Processor
QA	Quality Assurance
QC	Quality Control
RADM	Regional Acid Deposition Model
RCRA	Resource Conservation and Recovery Act
RAAS	Remedial Action Assessment System
RAGS	Risk Assessment Guidelines for Superfund
RAPS	Remedial Action Priority System
R&D	Research and Development
ReOpt	Remediation Options (remediation software)
RES	Office of Nuclear Regulatory Research
RESRAD	RESidual RADioactivity
RIP	early version of GoldSim software
SAS®	Statistical Analysis System
SEI	Software Engineering Institute
SMS	DoD's Surface Water Modeling System
SNF-EIS	Spent Nuclear Fuels Environmental Impact Statement
SQL	Structured Query Language
SSF	Site Simulation Files
S/U	Sensitivity/Uncertainty
SUM^3	Sensitivity/Uncertainty Multimedia Modeling Module

SWM	Stanford Watershed Model
TEDE	Total Effective Dose Equivalent
TMDL	Total Maximum Daily Load
TRIM	Total Risk Integrated Methodology
TRV	Toxicity Reference Value
TWRS	Tank Waste Remediation System
UDEP	Unified Data Exchange Protocol
UML	Unified Modeling Language
USACE	U.S. Corps of Engineers
USCM	Unified Conceptual Site Model
USDA	U.S. Department of Agriculture
USGS	U.S. Geological Survey
UTA	Unified Transport Approach
VAMP	VAlidation of Model Predictions
WERF	Water Environment Research Foundation
WES	Waterways Experiment Station (Army Corps of Engineers)
WIPP	Waste Isolation Pilot Plant
WMS	DoD's Watershed Modeling Systems

1.0 Introduction

U.S. Nuclear Regulatory Commission (NRC) staff from the Office of Nuclear Regulatory Research (NRC-RES) and the Office of Nuclear Materials Safety and Safeguards (NRC-NMSS) hosted an interagency workshop on multimedia environmental software and data systems on March 7–10, 2000, also referred to as the *March 2000* workshop. The environmental software systems that were discussed are used to evaluate contaminant release, transport and health effects through various media (e.g., air, ground, and surface water), and environmental pathways to human and ecological receptors. Because of limited resources and expanding modeling needs for environmental assessments, a need exists to share models, databases, and information technologies in new ways. A major motivation for the workshop was the desire of the participating Federal agencies to realize efficiencies and cost savings by using existing and future models, systems, and databases developed in their programs rather than developing totally new environmental-simulation software systems. The workshop participants brought together significant expertise, experiences, and modeling systems to begin the cooperative discussions. Federal agencies, their co-operators, and contractors participated in this inaugural gathering. The workshop agenda (see Appendix A) was developed over a period of many weeks to bring together the principal Federally sponsored programs in multimedia modeling. The workshop participants included model developers, model users, and Federal project managers responsible for developing and demonstrating the models' usefulness. The workshop focused on the issues of compatibility and linkage of multimedia models and systems as well as related environmental and health-effects databases. The following organizations participated in the planning of the workshop and/or sent attendees to the workshop:

- U.S. Nuclear Regulatory Commission
    - NRC-RES
    - NRC-NMSS
- U.S. Department of Energy (DOE)
    - Office of Environmental Management (EM)
    - Argonne National Laboratory (ANL)
    - Pacific Northwest National Laboratory (PNNL)
    - Oak Ridge National Laboratory (ORNL)
- U.S. Environmental Protection Agency (EPA)
    - Office of Radiation and Indoor Air (ORIA)
    - Office of Research and Development (ORD) at Athens (EPA-Athens)
    - Office of Solid Waste (OSW)
    - Office of Water (OW)
- U.S. Department of Defense (DoD), Army Corps of Engineers (USACE), Engineer Research and Development Center - Waterways Experiment Station (ERDC-WES)
- New Jersey Institute of Technology
- New Jersey Department of Environmental Protection
- Sandford Cohen & Associates
- Golder Associates, Inc.

1.1 Purpose

The purpose of this report is to describe the March 2000 workshop proceedings. In particular, the report identifies the participants and their affiliations (see Appendix B), captures the themes and discussions, and summarizes the principal outcomes and specific recommendations. The idea for this workshop originated one year ago during discussions at the "Public Workshop on Ground-Water Modeling Used in Dose Assessments," also held at NRC Headquarters, in June 1999. Before the workshop, the principal Federal Agencies and their contractors working on multimedia systems for environmental assessments were contacted and questioned about their interest and what presentations and discussions would be preferred, although the motivation for the collaborative effort identified at the workshop has been developing over a much longer time period. Draft agendas were formulated and sent to interested parties. Important secondary goals of the workshop, which were met, were to (1) summarize and document findings and (2) establish action items, including the interest in a second meeting.

1.2 Objectives of Workshop

The main objective of the workshop was to develop standard attributes for software systems that will link environmental/exposure/dose/risk models, disparate environmental databases, and modeling frameworks (systems) in a transparent manner, including web-based access and implementation from and on local and remote hardware and software. By meeting the objective, the design will establish a mechanism for different groups to link host (native) and remote (foreign) models and databases to disparate models and databases developed by others to support conceptual site-model development and risk/dose assessments.

1.3 Participant Objectives

This section describes the objectives of each of the participants and what they hoped to gain from the meeting in the context of multimedia modeling.

1.3.1 NRC – Research Objectives (Ralph Cady, NRC-RES)

From the perspective of waste-management and facility-decommissioning research, NRC recognizes the potential benefit from standardizing attributes for software systems linking environmental/exposure/dose/risk models, environmental databases, and modeling frameworks. The objectives of attending this workshop were to (1) gain from the experience of others in the assembled broad technical group concerned with environmental software compatibility and linkage, (2) develop a general preference for future development of attributes for environmental software compatibility and linkage, (3) identify and explore similar initiatives from diverse fields, and (4) consider future interactions and additional participants.

1.3.2 DOE – FRAMES Objectives (Paul Beam, DOE-EM)

DOE's EM office has supported the development and application of innovative environmental modeling systems for many years. One of these systems is the Framework for Risk Analysis in Multimedia Environmental Systems (FRAMES) developed by PNNL. DOE-EM will continue to support these types of systems that will facilitate DOE's future environmental analysis and decision processes. DOE-EM is also interested in better integrating environmental analysis and decision-support tools across DOE and other federal agencies. DOE-EM's objectives for attending the workshop were to

- support software-systems development that will facilitate DOE's future environmental analysis and decision processes
- provide a better understanding of DOE's future needs
- better integrate environmental-analysis and decision-support tools across DOE
- better integrate environmental-analysis and decision-support tools across Federal Agencies.

DOE-EM's desired attributes of integrated modeling systems are to

- Achieve Cost Savings
    - single-software platform with a suite of tools to allow tasks to be completed more efficiently and effectively
    - plug-and-play modules that allow appropriate models to be used in new applications
    - co-funded development efforts by multiple users
- Enhance Technical Credibility to Allow Use of Widely Accepted Models
    - allows focus of reviews to be on acceptance of any new models that meet desired objectives
    - helps overcome some of the "provincial" issues with technical acceptance of models
- Provide Better Consistency
    - common data specifications for modules
    - easy comparisons/benchmarking between models
    - standardized means of linking to other frameworks
    - consistent problem-definition protocols
- Improve Data Management
    - facilitate site and complex wide data management
    - allow use/access to current databases
    - add more tractability and accountability.

1.3.3 EPA – Models 2000 and Models 2001 Initiatives

The EPA has a mature and sophisticated rule-making infrastructure that is essential for developing its environmental programs. But if the overarching purpose for these programs is to maintain a healthy environment, then new decision-support tools are needed to ensure programmatic success. The EPA held a workshop in December 1997 to initiate the Models 2000 effort, with the goal to define improvements to EPA's environmental modeling capabilities and develop an implementation plan. This Agency-wide Models Implementation and Improvement Plan was expected to address the development, peer review and quality assurance/quality control (QA/QC), and application of environmental models. During the workshop, 11 action teams were established to perform the work: Quality Assurance and Peer Review Team, Modeling Paradigm Development Team, and 9 other teams.

The Quality Assurance and Peer Review Team prepared a handout on writing charters for modeling projects and products, which was included in Agency-wide Peer Review training conducted by the

Agency's Quality Staff. The purpose of the handout was to encourage peer review of models and to enhance staff use of the Agency's *Guidance for Conducting External Peer Review of Environmental Regulatory Models* (EPA 100-B-94-001). The team also developed a draft of *Guidance on Quality Assurance Project Plans for Modeling* that was to help those conducting modeling projects to meet Quality Assurance Project Plan requirements of the Agency's Directive EPA Order 5360.1 A2, *Policy and Program Requirements for the Mandatory Agency-wide Quality System*. Subsequently, the draft was revised by the Quality Staff and has recently undergone review by the Agency's Council on Regulatory Environmental Monitoring.

The Modeling Paradigm Development Team had 22 members, 15 representing EPA and 7 from other federal agencies and the private sector. They wrote the *Models 2000 Initiative: Software Development Vision and Goals*, held a Software Architecture Workshop, and built the WaterBeans[a] Integration Infrastructure prototype.

- The Models 2000 Initiative document includes a programmatic vision describing a new generation of integrated decision-support tools for managing environmental programs. The vision includes a 1) software vision that describes a common modeling framework, based on an expansive, open-source architecture and a product line of customer-based decision-support tools and 2) description of state-of-the-science software technologies, proven effective in other modeling domains, which can provide leverage in modernizing EPA modeling software and decision-support tools.

- The Software Architecture Workshop was held in April 1999 at EPA's National Exposure Research Laboratory (NERL). It provided an opportunity for EPA, U.S. Geological Survey (USGS), and other team members to collaborate with software engineers from the Software Engineering Institute (SEI) to become familiar with emerging architecture-based development processes that have evolved during a series of multimillion-dollar DoD software architecture research programs. The EPA Multimedia Integrated Modeling System (MIMS) architecture team was established by EPA software developers who attended this workshop.

- The WaterBeans Integration Infrastructure prototype was developed by members of the team to address the model integration problem. They developed a high-level software architecture that can support the integration of modeling software components at different levels of granularity, and produced a prototype called WaterBeans to test and evaluate the basic concepts underlying the architecture. WaterBeans may evolve, after a number of iterations, into an architecture that is robust enough to support some (or all) of the spatial scale and multimedia integrations needed in the common modeling framework. It currently has a limited set of modeling components, but it

  - provides the component integration to create new applications using either available components from existing models or newly designed enhanced components

  - will enable EPA or other model developers to leverage their investment in existing models by reimplementing these applications as WaterBeans compliant components

  - provides a set of principles (specifications) for developing new components

---

(a) WaterBeans is public domain software, developed by the Models 2000 Modeling Paradigm Development Team, with support from the EPA's Office of Wastewater Management.

- enables public domain and proprietary software components to run in the same application, mutually supporting one another

- demonstrates reusable code, in which the same components can work in either WaterBeans, existing applications (like SewerCAT or MMS), or new applications (such as MIMS)

- demonstrates the feasibility and benefits of using component-based software for urban drainage system modeling

- may enable EPA's air and water quality software to evolve into multimedia software.

The Modeling Paradigm Development Team obtained funding from the EPA Office of Wastewater Management to develop urban watershed decision-support tools, based on the technologies and product line of customer-based applications described in the Models 2000 Initiative. This software will be developed by NERL, and the project is scheduled to begin in Fiscal Year (FY) 2002. Other activities are described on the following website: www.epa.gov/ordntrnt/ORD/CREM.

During the Models 2000 effort, collaboration between EPA and other federal agencies on developing a unified, modular, common modeling framework and leveraging newer software technologies to modernize legacy code was one impetus that impelled the development of the Federal Agency Modeling Memorandum of Understanding (FAMMOU). FAMMOU has created a favorable climate for collaborative strategic planning and cooperative environmental modeling-software development. The primary objective of the Models 2001 Initiative is to integrate the Models 2000 effort and the FAMMOU implementation and to build the necessary partnerships to do so. As a result, the Water Environment Research Foundation (WERF) has adopted the key concepts in the Models 2000 Initiative and is establishing a new research focus area in environmental modeling to support developing the Initiative's common modeling framework. WERF is also working on a partnership vision, which will be included in the Initiative's revision, the Models 2001 Initiative.

1.3.4 EPA – Athens Objectives (Dave Brown/Gerry Laniak, EPA-ORD)

The Ecosystems Research Division of the NERL attended the March 2000 workshop for three reasons: (1) to provide input regarding technology attributes, (2) to determine overall degree of interest among the participants, and (3) to determine the level of commitment (time, personnel, finances) that may be required to participate in these activities into the future.

Some collaboration building objectives were to (1) communicate the importance of management in these endeavors and move toward a multi-agency MOU, and (2) investigate the possibilities of establishing specific collaborative efforts related to key issues, such as model-comparison studies, site-conceptualization protocols, and development of multimedia modeling-data sets for validation.

1.3.5 PNNL Objectives (John Buck, PNNL)

PNNL has extensive experience in creating innovative environmental modeling systems for government and industry applications. PNNL has developed FRAMES, which is a software platform being used by DOE, EPA, DoD, and industry to easily integrate independent environmental models into an integrated system for specific applications. PNNL's objectives for attending this workshop were to

- participate in establishing the "next generation" environmental modeling and decision-support communication protocols

- understand the technical-linkage needs of any systems that are developed in the future

- ensure that current and future PNNL projects are moving toward the "State of the Art" in system communication

- support the recommendations from this workshop

- strengthen working relationships with technical leads working on environmental modeling.

1.3.6 EPA – OSW Objectives (Stephen Kroner, EPA-OSW)

The OSW operates under the authority of the Resource Conservation and Recovery Act (RCRA) with a primary objective to protect human health and the environment by ensuring responsible national management of hazardous and nonhazardous waste. Our goals are to (1) conserve resources by reducing waste, (2) prevent future waste-disposal problems by writing result-oriented regulations, and (3) clean up areas where waste may have spilled, leaked, or been improperly disposed of. Much of this effort relies on estimating exposures and risk using fate/transport, uptake, exposure, and risk models. Since 1997, OSW and EPA's ORD have been developing an integrated, Multimedia, Multi-pathway, and Multiple Receptor Risk Assessment (3MRA) model to identify safe, constituent-specific exemption levels for low-risk hazardous wastes.

OSW's objectives for attending this workshop are to (1) share some of the experiences and lessons learned associated with designing, building, and populating a complex modeling tool, (2) identify areas that are currently problematic in the 3MRA, including evaluating multiple chemicals and sources simultaneously, improving the transparency of the model, and improving the visualization of the input and output data, and (3) understand where other groups are in the field and see if there are areas OSW could learn from these other groups.

1.3.7 EPA – ORIA Objectives (Chris Nelson/Dale Hoffmeyer/Tony Wolbarst, EPA-RIA)

ORIA is well aware that there are considerable differences among the various available environmental pathway modeling tools employed in the remediation of sites contaminated with radioactive materials; this can lead to inconsistent and even contradictory results, sometimes causing confusion and pointless disagreements among the regulatory agencies or between the agencies and the regulated community. The development of common platforms, such as FRAMES and the Dynamic Information Architecture System (DIAS), however, can contribute significantly toward the adoption of a coordinated and comprehensive methodology for carrying out scientifically sound and legally defensible site assessments. ORIA supports such efforts to improve the consistency and general effectiveness of modeling, and expects this workshop to provide a valuable opportunity for the sharing of good ideas.

1.3.8 ERDC – WES-ARAMS Objectives (Mark Dortch, ERDC-WES)

The objective of the Army Risk Assessment Modeling System (ARAMS) is to develop a computer-based decision-support system that integrates *multimedia* fate/transport, exposure, uptake, and effects of military-relevant compounds, including explosives and depleted uranium, to assess *human* and *ecological probabilistic* risks. The system should allow for both screening-level and comprehensive assessments. Although ARAMS is being developed for the Army, it is hoped that the system will be generally applicable to chemical-risk-assessment problems encountered by other services of the DoD, as well as other federal and state agencies. The objectives of attending this workshop were to (1) learn what other agencies are doing in this field, (2) learn how to leverage or benefit from others' developments, and (3) explore ways of working cooperatively with other agencies to link risk-assessment frameworks.

1.3.9 ERDC – WES-LMS Objectives (Jeff Holland, ERDC-WES)

ERDC is developing the Land Management System (LMS) to support decisions regarding the environmental quality of water and natural resources on both military installations and at USACE civil-works projects. Specific applications of LMS are anticipated to be environmental restoration, stewardship, and compliance as well as evaluating tradeoff in the planning and management for water and natural resources. The LMS is being developed as a web-based system with four interlaced functional levels: data level, modeling and simulation level, conceptual level, and the decision-support level. The objectives for ERDC participation in this workshop, from the perspective of the LMS, were to (1) explore common programming standards and information architectures between the differing systems represented by the workshop participants, (2) assess opportunities for synergism between workshop participants in the development of protocols and contracts for linkage of landscape models, geographic information systems (GISs), and various assessment and visualization tools, and (3) explore opportunities for developing standard computational objects and components by the differing workshop participants that, when made openly available, would greatly extend the scope and functionality of any of the systems represented within the workshop.

1.3.10 EPA-OAQPS Objectives (Brad Lyon, ORNL)

EPA's Office of Air Quality Planning and Standards (OAQPS) has the responsibility for the hazardous and criteria air-pollutant programs described by Sections 112 and 108 of the Clean Air Act (CAA). In 1996, OAQPS embarked on a multi-year effort to develop the Total Risk Integrated Methodology (TRIM), a time-series modeling system with multimedia capabilities for assessing human health and ecological risks from hazardous and criteria air pollutants. The TRIM design includes three modules: TRIM.FaTE (fate, transport, and ecological-exposure model), TRIM.Expo (human exposure event model) and TRIM.Risk (risk characterization model). Current collaborators with OAQPS on this project are EPA's ORD, Lawrence Berkeley National Laboratory, Oak Ridge National Laboratory, EC/R Incorporated, ICF Consulting, and MCNC-North Carolina Supercomputing Center. We have completed the first version of TRIM.FaTE, the multimedia fate and transport module, and are currently in the process of evaluating the TRIM.FaTE model, with application of this model by 2001. TRIM is being designed as an open-architecture system, specifically to facilitate the incorporation of new science and to integrate ORD modeling advances when available. Therefore, as part of attending this meeting, we hope to obtain a better understanding of the issues involved in linking models, as well as a clear picture of what we need to do to maintain compatibility with other models. It is critical that the TRIM project keep abreast of the latest software design movements in the environmental software community so that TRIM can properly take advantage of and be consistent with other models

1.3.11 State of New Jersey, Department of Environmental Protection (Bob Hazen)

A primary objective for attending the modeling workshop was to further uniformity and harmonization in modeling approaches, which can be applied to a wide variety of regulatory purposes. A particular need for multimedia models is to proportionally allocate the importance of different environmental sources of the same chemical agent to a particular receptor. Atmospheric deposition, direct discharges to surface water, historic sediment contamination, and groundwater to surface migration of chemicals from hazardous waste sites all contribute to fish contamination in New Jersey estuaries. It is also of interest to automate a modeling analysis of all these sources using available GIS landscape data, which currently exist in great detail for the region of concern. The construction of a comprehensive environmental modeling approach would help determine exactly which data are necessary in the periodic data submissions from the regulated community. The goal of a seamless transition through acquiring, storing, retrieving, and analyzing data would be aided by a detailed advanced knowledge of the modeling strategy. Another objective is to use multimedia models in state university environmental science programs as a means to knit together air pollution, hydrology, soil science, and environmental health curricula.

1.4 Definition of Terms Used in the Workshop

Definitions of terms typically used during the workshop are presented as follows.

- **Architecture** – Architecture contains four components, described as follows:

    1. Data Architecture – Data Architecture refers to the data structure required to perform activities, including data administration requirements.

2. Hardware Architecture – Hardware Architecture refers to the physical environment (servers, routers, cables, etc.) required to perform activities.

3. Security Architecture – Security Architecture refers to security processes and rules, including remote access, password rotation, and anti-virus procedures.

4. Software Architecture – Software Architecture refers to the software environment required to perform activities.

- **Attributes** – Attributes are characteristics and behaviors that a piece of software must possess to function adequately for its intended purpose. An attribute is often called a requirement, and a good attribute is testable.

- **Components** – Components of the system represent those elements that are housed within or accessed by the system, which facilitates communication between elements. The components need to have the capability to exist and independently operate, where appropriate, outside of the system. Models and databases represent typical components.

- **Design** – A design is a comprehensive description of how a piece of software will function (i.e., how it will meet its attributes).

- **Input** – Input is information or data transferred or to be transferred from a producing medium to a consuming medium—any data/information that are required to process a model (output from one model may be input to another). Input can be provided through a variety of structures, including database format (flat or relational), manual entry, and parameter files.

- **Model/Code** – Loosely defined herein to represent the software product for simulating the release, fate and transport, exposure, intake, or risk/hazard of chemicals released into the environment; however, a model/code can simulate any phenomena and is not limited to hazardous waste site assessments.

- **Module** – A module is a Model/Code and accompanying (1) pre- and post-processors for communicating with other models, databases, frameworks, etc., and (2) model-specific user interface (MUI).

- **Output** – Output is computer results (e.g., answers to mathematical problems; statistical, analytical, or accounting figures; or production schedules) or information transferred from a producing medium to a consuming medium. Output is any data/information that are provided as a result of processing a model (output from one model may be input to another). Output can be provided in different structures including databases (flat and relational) or graphical.

- **Ownership** – The "owner" (1) controls the software or database, (2) is responsible for its QA/QC, modifications, documentation, and upkeep, and (3) limits access by others.

- **Process** – Process is a generic term that may include compute, assemble, compile, interpret, and generate. Herein, it refers to the transformation of input data into output data.

- **Specifications** – Specifications are detailed descriptions of an interface to a computer program or set of subroutines such that another programmer could develop a program that would make proper use to the subroutines.

- **System or Framework** – Loosely defines a linked grouping of models, modules, databases, processors, or combination. The System or Framework represents software that coordinates the interaction and communication of components (models and databases) that comprise the system and is independent of the components that comprise the system. For the system to be independent of the components, the components need to have the capability to exist and independently operate, where appropriate, outside of the system. The protocols or specifications, which define how components communicate, are considered part of the system.

- **Testable** – Refers to the property of having the capability to examine and interrogate, such that a clear and concise conclusion can be drawn.

- **Trusteeship** – A "trustee" administers the use of software or a database; ensures *shared responsibility* between those who own the software or database; is responsible for its QA/QC, modifications, documentation, upkeep; and allows access by others.

1.5 Subsequent Activities Derived from the Workshop

1.5.1 Merging 3MRA and FRAMES-V1

PNNL, under the guidance and direction of EPA and DOE, developed the software technology system titled FRAMES. As a natural extension of the joint effort between DOE and EPA, EPA instructed PNNL to refine and extend FRAMES to build a technology software-modeling system capable of conducting a national assessment of exposure and risk due to contaminant releases from hazardous waste sites. This effort was to support the promulgation of rules associated with the Hazardous Waste Identification Rule (HWIR), using the 3MRA methodology.

The primary objective is to design and implement enhancements to the FRAMES and 3MRA modeling technologies. FRAMES and 3MRA, while conceptually similar, are different in two fundamental ways. First, the manner in which data are managed in 3MRA is more advanced relative to FRAMES. Second, FRAMES was designed to facilitate site-specific assessments and thus has a user interface for collecting data from the user. The 3MRA system was designed to facilitate a national assessment and thus does not contain a site-specific user interface. The enhancements center on merging the best features of the existing 3MRA technology with the existing FRAMES technology and advancing the data-exchange protocols.

The initial step for combining 3MRA and FRAMES was to develop and document attributes for a unified system, a unified CSM, and a DEP. A CSM represents a simplified description of the environmental problem to be modeled. A DEP defines how data are transferred and exchanged between components (e.g., modules, databases, frameworks). Attributes are characteristics and behaviors that a piece of software must possess to function adequately for its intended purpose. The purpose of these attributes is to state those conditions that define the merger between FRAMES – Version 1 and the 3MRA software. The attributes outlined in Chapter 5 formed the basis for developing attributes associated with the merger of these two systems, attributes that are subsequently presented in Chapter 6.

1.5.2 Memorandum of Understanding

Six Federal agencies have agreed to work together on research and development (R&D) for multimedia (air, groundwater, surface water, etc.) environmental models used to assess contaminant risks to human populations by formerly signing a Memorandum of Understanding (MOU) in July 2001. A copy of the final MOU, as signed by the original six Federal agencies, is presented in Appendix F. The six charter agencies include

1. EPA, NERL

2. USACE, Engineering Research Development Center (ERDC, formerly the Waterways Experiment Station in Vicksburg, Mississippi)

3. USGS, Waterways Research Division, U.S. Department of Interior

4. DOE, Environmental Management

5. Agricultural Research Service (ARS), U.S. Department of Agriculture

6. NRC, Office of Research.

Other organizations that have expressed interest in the effort include

- Natural Resources Conservation Service (formerly the Soil Conservation Service), U.S. Department of Agriculture
- National Oceanic and Atmospheric Administration, U.S. Department of Commerce
- Cooperative State Research Education and Extension Service
- Bureau of Reclamation.

Informal discussions began among DOE, NRC, and EPA—and later the Defense Department—in 1995. In March 2000, NRC hosted a workshop on *Environmental Software Systems Compatibility and Linkage.* Federal agencies and private-sector representatives attended and were enthusiastic about the possibilities identified in the workshop, as outlined in this document, and called for a more formal, ongoing effort. The workshop ended with agreement on a recommendation that the relationship among the Federal agencies involved in the workshop should be formalized and that "no one agency or group should be 'in charge' of this collaborative effort"; rather, it should be a collaboration of equals working toward a unified system.

The MOU establishes a framework for cooperation and coordination among the participants in R&D of multimedia environmental models, software, and related databases. Participants have a strong interest in both framework models and in the underlying science. Activities covered by the MOU can include development, enhancements and applications, and assessments of site-specific, generic, and process-oriented multimedia environmental models. The Agencies intend for the MOU to provide a mechanism for them to pursue common technology in multimedia environmental modeling with a shared technology basis. This does not mean that the Agencies are trying to develop a single, multi-agency model. The Agencies are trying to obtain mutual benefits from R&D programs and ensure effective information exchanges between their respective staff and contractors. The R&D programs include "development and field applications of a wide variety of software modules, data processing tools, and uncertainty-assessment approaches for understanding and predicting contaminant transport processes, including the impact of chemical and non-chemical stressors on human and ecological health." The Agencies will

- promote technical coordination
- identify joint R&D programs of mutual interest and sources of funding. The MOU specifically states that Agencies are not agreeing to commit resources, other than individual participants, by participating in the MOU)
- assist in arranging for supplementary inter-agency R&D agreements
- facilitate the coordination and exchange of R&D data and technical information.

Because of Federal Advisory Committee Act requirements, full participation is limited to Federal agencies; however, foreign and international agencies, as well as private-sector representatives, can serve as consultants and advisors.

2.0 Historical Perspective, and Workshop Structure and Process

Prepared by Gene Whelan and Tom Nicholson

2.1 Historical Perspective

Over the past 35 years, medium-specific models have been and will continue to be developed in an effort to understand and predict environmental phenomena, including fluid-flow patterns (e.g., groundwater, surface water, and air), contaminant migration and fate, human or wildlife exposures, impacts from specific toxicants to specific species and their organs, cost-benefit analyses, impacts from remediation alternatives, etc. The evolution of multiple-media assessment tools has followed a logical progression (Whelan et al. 1997):

- In 1959, the Stanford Watershed Model (SWM) was developed. It represented one of the first integrated models as it linked multiple processes by simulating the land phase of the hydrologic cycle for an entire watershed.

- In 1969, ORNL presented the Unified Transport Approach (UTA), which coupled (hard-wired) detailed numerical models, describing individual environmental media (e.g., groundwater, air, surface water, and soil). Because (1) the models were difficult to understand, operate, modify, and maintain, (2) data for operating the models were generally unavailable, and, most importantly, (3) computer power to drive the system was lacking at the time, the UTA did not progress into general use.

- In 1984, the first fully coupled sequential multimedia model, which accounted for temporally and spatially varying contamination within designated media, was introduced. Each medium-specific model was "hard-wired" into the system, so replacing medium-specific components was not built into the system. These multimedia models were made possible with the introduction of desk-top computing.

- Around 1990, the development of large multi-purpose frameworks began, which "hard-wired" a suite of codes together and investigated, not just the distribution of contaminants in the environment, but relationships between a suite of issues deemed valuable (regulatory criteria, data quality objectives, Comprehensive Environmental Response, Compensation, and Liability Act (CERCLA), RCRA processes, etc.).

- In 1995, multimedia frameworks, which link disparate models and databases together in a "Plug & Play" atmosphere while maintaining the integrity of legacy codes and databases, were first being designed.

Estimates of chemical fate and transport used in support of environmental regulatory activities have been for the most part determined with single-medium models. Major federal environmental statutes (CAA, Clean Water Act, RCRA, CERCLA) have resulted in state regulations with program-administrative structures for a single medium. Environmental measurement, engineering compliance requirements, and enforcement strategies are essentially self-contained in air, water, and land. While RCRA and CERCLA have guidance with provisions for multimedia modeling, the

2.1

modeling approaches do not necessarily maintain mass balance. Triggers for health risk are in concentration and not mass units.

There have been recent federal and state environmental initiatives that are inherently multimedia in approach. The interest is to estimate the combined effects of multiple sources of multiple chemical toxic agents. The reason for the initiatives is that information derived from the current suite of regulatory statutes is not adequate to answer the questions posed. Data are often recorded in numerous incompatible systems because use for multimedia analysis is neither required nor anticipated. Watershed toxics analysis and comparative risk are two efforts that attempt to resolve multiple source, multiple chemical-exposure questions. One objective of watershed projects has been to determine strategies to reduce potential human health risk due to accumulation of toxic metals and organics in fish. An answer to this question involves modeling air, soil, water, and sediment sources to fish biomass while maintaining mass balance with the source terms involved. Comparative risk is another initiative, which has resulted in federal and state efforts to summarize the exposure and risk to people from various documented sources described in air, soil, water, and food. For the most part, single-medium models and the data collected in compliance with laws conceived in single-medium terms do not provide sufficient information regarding the relative importance of different source terms to overall human exposure. This is in part because intermedia transport, if considered at all, is estimated in one direction only. For chemicals that do not strongly partition in a single medium, there may be significant flux back to the medium of origin before advective processes remove it from the system.

The current risk paradigm (e.g., CERCLA and RCRA) follows the life of a chemical from source to receptor. Multiple models and approaches have been developed to address this paradigm, many duplicating the effort of others and some representing new innovative and creative solutions. The next step in the development process is to ensure that the technical community comes together to enhance communication and technology transfer. As such, this workshop was held to discuss ways to develop standard attributes for software systems that will allow for remote or local communication of environmental/exposure/dose/risk models, disparate environmental databases, and modeling frameworks (systems) in a transparent manner, including web-based access and implementation from and on local and remote hardware and software. By meeting the objective, various designs could establish a mechanism for different groups to link host (i.e., native) and remote (foreign) models and databases to disparate models and databases developed by others to support conceptual site-model development and risk/dose assessments.

By meeting this objective, it is hoped that when modifications to the standard risk paradigm occurs, the technical community will be prepared to respond in a cogent and responsive manner. For example, a scientific shift is underway to also follow the life cycle of a human and the potential impacts to chemical exposure along that life-cycle path. The human life cycle is, in effect, orthogonal to a path that a chemical might follow, where these paths will periodically cross for different chemicals and humans under different situations. As such, software developed to understand the life cycle of one could be used to understand the life cycle of the other. This workshop represents a first step in developing software protocols that bridge these gaps.

2.2 Workshop Structure and Process

The workshop was structured to facilitate meaningful dialogue on both broad multimedia modeling themes (e.g., model and framework connectivity, web-based access, and information architecture), and specific application examples. The workshop brought together scientists and engineers in the Federal community and their contractors who truly have an interest in ensuring communication between environmental software products. An important assumption was that technical problems would not be solved at the first meeting, but it would begin a discourse for mapping out approaches to solving them. It was important for the interested parties to discuss their objectives and expectations. This first workshop provided an excellent opportunity for introductions and networking.

The workshop agenda, which is presented in Appendix A, was designed to address the workshop objective by incorporating input and feedback from the participants; hence, the agenda represented a living document until the time of the workshop. The workshop was three-days in length with a set-up day that preceded the workshop and a summary day that succeeded the workshop. The set-up day provided the participants an opportunity to load their software on to NRC computers, which were demonstrated on the third day of the workshop. The middle 3 days were set aside for the more "formal" meeting. The day succeeding the workshop was set aside to provide time to begin the process of compiling the summary manuscript, documenting the activities of the workshop and outlining action items and the next meeting (if appropriate).

Day 1 of the workshop allowed participants an opportunity to introduce themselves and state their objectives. Because the main objective is to develop standard attributes, protocols, and specifications for linking environmental/exposure/dose/risk models, disparate environmental databases, and modeling frameworks (systems) in a transparent manner, the afternoon of Day 1 focused on attributes of software that allow for communication and linkage. The science underlying the software systems was not the focus, but rather the capability of the software system to facilitate development and application of the science. Four working groups were established to independently develop software attributes. In the morning of Day 2, each of the participants was provided an opportunity to present his/her software concepts, which represented insight as to where the current technology is. The intent was to be as succinct and focused as possible and to outline what has already been developed so the software world is not reinvented. In the afternoon, each group facilitator reviewed his/her attribute lists. During the morning of Day 3, the group convened to discuss each attribute and develop a composite and finalized list as to the software requirements necessary to promote communication between current software and the development of disparate software tools and databases to support release/transport/exposure/risk assessments. Finally, for those interested in seeing demonstrations of some of the software, software demonstrations were held during the afternoon of the third day.

3.0 Motivation for Risk Assessment Framework Development

Prepared by J. Holland and M. Dortch

For more than 20 years, risk assessments have addressed the simulated contaminant release, fate and transport, exposure, and risk for a single chemical within a single environmental medium. Currently, government agencies are in the process of developing and implementing computer-based tools that view the environment from multiple dimensions, accounting for various waste forms, environmental media, and relationships between the waste sites and the surrounding sensitive receptors. These computer-based tools are physics- and PC-based, integrated methodologies that view the environment from a more holistic, systematic viewpoint (Laniak et al. 1997; Mills et al. 1997). Tables 3.1 and 3.2 illustrate the evolving increase in complexity associated with risk assessment and the dimensionality involved in simulating environmental systems, respectively (Whelan and Laniak 1998).

Table 3.1. EPA Regulatory Focus (After Whelan and Laniak 1998)

PAST Singe Pathway Analysis	PRESENT Multiple Pathway Analysis	FUTURE Integrated Systems Analysis
Single Chemical	Multiple Chemicals	Mixture/Speciation/Microbiology
Multiple Chemical Sources	Multiple Chemical Sources	Multiple Chemical/Nonchemical Stressors
Single Medium Fate & Transport	Linked Media Fate & Transport	Integrated Multimedia Fate & Transport with Mass Balance and Feedback
Single Exposure Route	Multiple Exposure Route Analysis	Integrated Exposure Route Analysis
Primary Human Health	Chemical/Exposure-Route Specific Risk	Aggregated Risk to Human Populations and Ecological Systems
Qualitative Uncertainty	Quantitative Uncertainty	Quantitative Uncertainty

There are motivating factors to design more comprehensive risk-based frameworks that can account for increasingly complex modeling systems. First, there is a need to assess risks in an increasingly complex and realistic manner, involving multiple disciplines. Second, there is a need to be consistent across levels of assessments (screening to detailed). The concept of a software-based modeling platform allows for both screening and complex models to be developed and applied within a single modeling system. In such a system, the logical link between first-step screening analyses and more complex assessments is clear. Finally, there is a need for efficient collection and use of data. The systematic approach associated with a tiered assessment ensures that data collected and used in a screening-level analysis is consistent with that used in the more detailed assessment.

Table 3.2. Dimensions of Exposure and Research Questions (After Whelan and Laniak 1998)

SPATIAL	local, regional, global
TEMPORAL	short-term/acute, seasonal, long-term/chronic
CHEMICAL	organics (pesticides, dioxin, furans, HCH, PAHs, PCBs, etc.), inorganics (organo-metals, lead, cadmium, mercury, tin, etc.)
ENVIRONMENTAL MEDIA	air, water (precipitation, groundwater, surface water), soil, sediment, biota (food chain)
ENVIRONMENTAL SETTINGS	agricultural, industrial, residential
CHEMICAL/ ECOLOGICAL FATE CHARACTERISTICS	Speciation, reactivity, degradability, volatility, phase equilibrium constants, complexation, bioaccumulation, biomagnification
ENVIRONMENTAL TRANSPORT AND TRANSFER	advection, dispersion, deposition, washout, degradation, partitioning, erosion, runoff, volatilization, suspension, sedimentation
RECEPTORS	human (children, occupation sensitive, general population), wildlife (fish, birds, reptiles, mammals)
EXPOSURE ROUTES	inhalation (gases, particulates), ingestion (plant, meat, milk, aquatic food, water, soil), dermal contact, external dose (radionuclides)
RISK END POINTS	human (cancer, non-cancer), ecological (individual, species, communities, habitats)

Each of the government agencies has and intends to use multimedia assessment modeling tools to help assist them in performing various aspects of risk assessments from site-specific, installation-wide, or national perspectives. This section overviews the requirements motivating the development and use of multimedia tools and frameworks for the various groups that attended the workshop.

3.1 Motivation for EPA Multimedia Assessment Tools

The National Research Council, in a recent review of significant emerging scientific issues, has identified improved models of pollutant transport and transformation and more effective risk-assessment methodologies as examples of core research areas that are needed to support problem-driven research across EPA programs (NRC 1997). Tables 3.3 and 3.4 summarize the increasing number of programs and activities across EPA that require a multimedia assessment of human and/or ecological exposure and risk. In response to this increased emphasis on multimedia risk assessment, EPA's ORD has begun to formulate unified and integrated approaches to develop and deliver the science and engineering involved in multimedia-based exposure and risk assessment. Fundamental to this effort is the design and implementation of modeling-based technologies, including environmental databases and models along with a wide variety of data-analysis tools (GIS, data visualization, etc.). Future efforts to provide the necessary technologies will be constrained by a shrinking budget and will be challenged by the need for scientific consistency across the assessment landscape. For these reasons, the EPA-ORD is interested in establishing collaborative relationships with the larger community of multimedia model developers both within the EPA and other Federal Agencies.

Table 3.3. National Multimedia Programs/Activities[b]

Responsible EPA Office	Programs/Activities with Significant Multimedia Aspects
Office of Air and Radiation	Hazardous Air Pollutant Program Electric Utility Hazardous Air Pollutant Study Section 112 Risk Assessments to Support Maximum Achievable Control Technology Standards CAA Regulations Disposal of Low-Level Radioactive Waste
Office of Enforcement and Compliance Assurance	Multimedia Enforcement, National Enforcement Screening Strategy
Office of Prevention, Pesticides, and Toxic Substances	New Chemicals Program Endocrine Disruption Research Initiative
ORD	Combustor Emissions Ecological and Human Health Exposure Evaluations Industrial-Solvents Replacements
Office of Solid Waste and Emergency Response (OSWER)	Municipal Solid Waste Landfill Rule Toxic Characteristics Program Hazardous Waste Characteristics Scoping Study Hazardous Waste Identification Rule Hazardous Waste Listing Evaluations Hazardous Waste Delisting RCRA Hazardous Waste No-Migration Petitions Superfund Lead Exposure/Lead Cleanup Regulations
OW	Wellhead Protection Program Underground Injection Control, Land-Disposal Restrictions Disposal of Municipal Sewage Sludge National Watershed Assessment Project

---

(b) HydroGeologic. 1998. *Characterization of Multimedia-Based Regulatory Activities.* Prepared by HydroGeologic Inc. for the U.S. Environmental Protection Agency, National Exposure Research Laboratory, Ecosystems Research Division, Office of Research and Development, Athens, Georgia (Draft).

Table 3.3 (Contd)

Responsible EPA Office	Programs/Activities with Significant Multimedia Aspects
Office of Air and Radiation, Office of Prevention, Pesticides, and Toxic Substances, OSWER	Source-Reduction Review Project
EPA, Agency-Wide	Common Sense Initiative Environmental Technology Initiative Program Reinvention for Innovative Technology (Refit) Program (under Environmental Technology Initiative Program) Reinvention for Multimedia Permitting High Performance Computing and Communications Program, Environmental Modeling
Toxic Substances and Hazardous Waste Subcommittee, National Science and Technology Council, Executive Office	National R&D Strategy for Toxic Substances and Hazardous and Solid Waste
International Organization for Standardization	ISO 14001, International Environmental Management System Standards

Table 3.4. Regional/State Multimedia Programs/Activities[a]

Responsible EPA Office	Programs/Activities with Significant Multimedia Aspects
ORD	Regional-Scale Air Toxics Modeling
Office of Solid Waste and Emergency Response (administered by EPA Regions and States)	Brownfields
Chesapeake Bay Program Office, EPA Region 3	Chesapeake Bay Program Airborne Nox Reduction
Great Lakes National Program Office	Great Lakes Water Quality Initiative, Great Lakes National Program
Long Island Sound Office, EPA Regions 1 and 2	National Estuary Program, Long Island Sound Study
EPA Region 8	Ecosystem Protection Initiative
EPA Region 10	Regional Comparative Risk Project and Priority Basin Performance Plan

(a) HydroGeologic. 1998. *Characterization of Multimedia-Based Regulatory Activities.* Prepared by HydroGeologic Inc. for the U.S. Environmental Protection Agency, National Exposure Research Laboratory, Ecosystems Research Division, Office of Research and Development, Athens, Georgia (Draft).

3.2 Motivation for DOE Multimedia Assessment Tools

With more than 36 major installations across the country—containing a variety of wastes (e.g., organics, metals, solvents, radionuclides, and mixed wastes), waste streams (liquid, semi-solid, solid), and waste types (solid waste, tanks, contaminated sediments, air, surface waters, vadose zones, aquifers, etc.)—DOE has one of the most complex and diverse sets of environmental problems to deal with as a result of the Cold War and its legacy. The diversity and complexity of these problems are well illustrated by the support programs that are being developed to address the need for sound scientific tools and approaches. DOE has performed a number of installation- and complex-wide assessments. Installation-wide assessments have included the following:

- DOE's Hanford Remedial Action Environmental Impact Statement (HRA-EIS), which evaluated and integrated the impacts associated with 1200 past-practice waste sites for 150 constituents, for four land-use options, to an 80-km radius (DOE 1994).

- DOE's Hanford Tank Waste Remediation System (TWRS), which evaluated and integrated the impacts associated with 237 tanks containing 177 million curies in 212 million liters to an 80-km radius (DOE/DOE 1996).

- Single-Shell Tank Release and Exposure/Risk Assessments, which (1) evaluated public-health impacts for the Hanford high-level waste tanks (Buck et al. 1995), (2) prepared waste-characterization plans (Droppo et al. 1991), and (3) provided design and characterization recommendations for closure decisions (Buck et al. 1991).

Complex-Wide assessments have included the following:

- DOE's Baseline EM Report (BEMR), which evaluated DOE's environmental waste problems from a life-cycle assessment perspective (Gelston et al. 1995).

- DOE's Programmatic Environmental Impact Statement (PEIS), which performed a preliminary risk evaluation of DOE's complex-wide waste sites.

- Spent Nuclear Fuels Environmental Impact Statement (SNF-EIS), which investigated options for stabilizing, transporting, and storing all portions of DOE-owned SNF, except for K-Basin SNF (DOE 1995a, Whelan et al. 1994).

- K-Basin Environmental Impact Statement (K-Basin EIS), which investigated options for stabilizing, transporting, and storing K Basin SNF (DOE 1995b).

- Molybdenum-99 Environmental Impact Statement (Moly 99 EIS), which investigated options for producing molybdenum-99 to provide medical needs in the nuclear medicine and diagnostic arena (DOE 1995c).

- DOE's Environmental Survey, which performed DOE's first preliminary risk evaluation of DOE's complex-wide waste sites.

Environmental-assessment modeling tools developed in the last decade give DOE critical information on potential risk and benefits of environmental operations and management. While most tools are focused on a single aspect of the environment, such as air-pollutant dispersion, surface-water discharges, or groundwater contamination, this results in incomplete answers to key environmental issues. Additionally, many integrated tools are constrained to analyze only one environmental medium, limiting their application and usability. Even the best-integrated models in the world are useless without clear and useful display of the massive information created by models. Easily understandable and reportable information from these models is paramount for decision-makers.

Flexible and holistic approaches are needed to understand how industrial activities affect humans and the environment. These approaches should incorporate models that integrate across scientific disciplines, allow tailored solutions for specific activities, and provide meaningful information to business and technical managers. The key is identifying, analyzing, and managing potential Environment, Safety, and Health risks. Multimedia tools would help to provide a consistent set of approaches to not only meet these needs, but also to meet similar needs that DOE will experience at its installations. As illustrated by past complex-wide assessments, these multimedia tools would support priority setting and budget decisions.

3.3 Motivation for NRC Multimedia Assessment Tools

The NRC staff uses multimedia environmental-assessment codes for reviewing license amendments for decommissioning and waste-disposal activities. The codes are used to review the licensees' conceptual models, evaluate various possible environmental pathways, and assess parameter inputs. The NRC staff reviews of the licensee's technical-basis documents and their confirmatory analyses serve as a basis for license determinations.

For example, the NRC staff and its contractors have developed a methodology for calculating doses to demonstrate compliance with the radiological criteria for decommissioning and license termination as documented in NUREG-1549 "Decision Methods for Dose Assessment to Comply with Radiological Criteria for License Termination" (NRC 1998). The environmental pathways include both air and water, focusing on doses due to exposure, inhalation, and ingestion of residual radioactivity. Detailed information on the development and implementation of the dose-assessment methodology for decommissioning reviews is provided in the NUREG/CR-5512 technical series reports.

3.4 Motivation for DoD Multimedia Assessment Tools

DoD has a broad range of user requirements and problem types motivating its development and use of multimedia modeling, assessment, and framework tools:

- training lands management
- contaminated military site cleanup
- testing-range management and stewardship
- deposition of airborne contaminants (due to live firing) and their fate in the environment
- chemical/biological threat assessment

- wetland permit evaluations
- coastal-zone management
- watershed management and restoration
- aquatic-ecosystem restoration
- dredging operations

It should be noted that many of the same issues motivating others within this workshop to use and develop multimedia frameworks are of importance to DoD. For example, the movement of contaminants through integrated atmospheric, surface water, groundwater, and overland transport mechanisms is key to assessing both risk and optimal cleanup strategies at multiple military installations. However, it should also be noted that these same multimedia pathways are key to restoring major aquatic and terrestrial ecosystems whose hydro-periods or water quality have been impacted by anthropogenic activities. Further, the integration of multiple media (particularly surface water -groundwater interaction with overland flow) is essential to managing watershed-scale and wetland water resources.

Three specific areas of DoD multimedia assessment are presented below. Note again that the term "multimedia" is applied at its broadest scale—that is, the consideration of flow, constitutive transport, and risk (whether it is human or ecological in nature) through multiple-media types.

3.4.1 Military Installation Environmental Quality

The resource-management issues facing U.S. military installations range from contaminated groundwater/soil cleanup to erosion and storm-water control, dust control, protection of historic and prehistoric sites, and threatened and endangered species habitat. As an example, DoD has thousands of sites on its military installations that are requiring or will require some level of remediation. Issues of both human and ecological health are of concern. The predominant technologies being used to address these issues include GIS, multi-dimensional, multi-component groundwater and surface-water modeling (to delineate exposure pathways and to optimize cleanup strategies), and risk assessment. Installation of spatial information, such as the location of man-made features (roads, utilities, firing/testing ranges, contaminant sources), and natural features (terrain, vegetation, soils) is being managed through GIS. As a natural extension of this use of GIS, there is a growing requirement for modeling and analysis output to be provided in multiple formats, including those compatible with GIS ingest. Animation and multi-dimensional graphics are used for installation resource issues (particularly for installation cleanup), but much less so than GIS technologies. Analyses have a predictive nature for periods ranging from days to decades. Long-term analysis tools range from low order (e.g., one or zero dimensional, often steady state), highly-parameterized solutions to fully three-dimensional analyses based on first principles equations. The use of the differing technologies is highly uncoupled, and there are only limited linkages between the disparate technologies to facilitate their integrated use.

3.4.2 Major Aquatic Ecosystems

Chesapeake Bay is one of the United States' most productive estuarine ecosystems. The use of technology for Chesapeake Bay is representative of analogous situations for the South Florida Ecosystem, the Upper Mississippi River System, the San Diego Bay, Columbia/Snake River System, San Francisco Bay, and a host of additional large-scale water-resource investigations of national importance. A broad-based partnership, made up of Chesapeake Bay state agencies, the EPA, USACE, and many additional partners, has been studying the effectiveness of a variety of management alternatives for improving the health of Bay. Highly-sophisticated, predictive three-dimensional hydrodynamic and water quality modeling, lumped-parameter watershed modeling, GIS, extensive field data collection and management, and other technologies are being used within the Bay community to assess the movement of nutrients and contaminants through multiple media. Recently, higher trophic-level modeling and assessment have also been introduced. Tradeoff analyses (e.g., "what-if analyses") are being conducted to evaluate potential long-term (e.g., decadal) impacts of decision making before implementation. Differing modeling and analysis technologies are being used primarily in an uncoupled fashion (e.g., watershed modeling is conducted to provide inputs to estuarine modeling, hydrodynamic modeling provides inputs to water-quality modeling, etc.) with GIS and visualization tools accessing these and other data for presentation purposes. Human-in-the-loop controls are required to process output from one analysis tool for input to a second tool, GIS, or visualization. Collaborative use of the products from these analyses within the Bay community is augmented by developing a variety of multi-dimensional animation and graphical components that are shared through onsite meetings, web-site-information posting and interrogation, and email. A wide range of users, including scientists, political decision makers, and the public, exists within the Bay community.

3.4.3 Watershed Analyses

Increasingly, planners and land managers are assessing resource decision making at the watershed scale because of the natural integration of processes that occurs at that scale. Agricultural and urban watershed investigations are underway to assess new agricultural practices, total maximum daily loadings, local and urban flood control, ecosystem management, and tradeoffs in land use both spatially and temporally for multiple purposes. Watershed modeling tools covering flow, nutrient and water quality constitutive transport, sediment transport, and contaminant transport have been in use in varying levels of sophistication for several decades. These tools have been packaged in integrated computational systems that provide single point-of-access to the models, parameter-estimation techniques, data-management methods, visualization, and a host of graphical and tabular outputs. Recently, investigations in this area have moved toward real-time analyses as well as planning scenario studies. An example of such real-time analyses is warnings for flash flooding. However, significant improvements in data-model and model-model connectivity, seamless data flow, and model reliability are required. As an example, the U.S. Army's Hydrologic Engineering Center, a leading developer of modeling and analysis tools for water management, is only now providing for interoperability (seamless connectivity) among the differing models, analytical tools, and data sources for its family of riverine and watershed modeling and analysis capabilities.

3.5   Motivation for Multimedia Assessment Tools to Support State Activities

State government statutes and regulations are directly responsible for many monitoring and enforcement activities, which result in control of the flow of toxic chemicals into the environment. The legal structure and resulting programmatic function often constrain the use of multimedia and multi-source chemical fate and transport analysis. The current legal framework for government action needs to be analyzed for the potential efficiencies inherent in multimedia analytic tools. The details of state decision making are based on rules established in the process agency's interpretation of the language in the controlling federal statutes and the regional regulatory context. For example, remedial alternatives for waste sites are developed from a site analysis, which in part depends on the predicted transport of toxic chemicals to human receptors and an estimate of health risk. Many states have tailored superfund guidance specifically for regional landscape conditions, such as rainfall and the general proximity of water bodies. However, property boundaries of the site in question often limit the scope of the investigation, and it is not extended to other sites in the immediate area to determine aggregate exposure and health effects. Air sources and deposition are not considered in the management of hazardous site cases if they do not originate with the responsible party, and the contribution of land sources is not generally considered in point-source air-risk assessments.

The result of the single media, one-source-at-a-time regulatory approach is that in areas with numerous sources side by side, it is possible for every source to be in compliance while the exposure resulting from all of them may exceed benchmark concentrations. There are some regulatory approaches, such as the Total Daily Maximum Loads (TMDLs) and environmental justice initiatives, that are more likely candidates for multimedia analysis. TMDL determination inherently integrates multiple sources for the large land areas associated with watersheds. Environmental justice evaluation calls for the summing of multiple sources of potential toxic chemical exposure to estimate community risk. Because both of these programs involve an analysis of sources that arise in multiple media, which must be summed, they are inherently more receptive to multimedia-modeling methods than regulations driven by point sources.

Sorting out the single-media modeling output as obtained from various regulatory programs so that aggregate or spatially or temporally resolved predicted media concentrations are available is probably impossible. This means that the relative importance or competing sources cannot be determined. A better approach would involve cross-communicating single-medium models or a comprehensive multimedia model used as the backbone for regulatory activities in all environmental media. Unconnected multimedia models applied to single media sources can also cause problems. EPA's OSWER Combustor guidance and Superfund guidance each move chemicals through multiple-media pathways, but by different algorithms. For example, the relationship between air and soil concentrations of the same chemical will be different in the different multimedia models. These contradictions do not become a noticeable problem until regulatory efforts start to overlap spatially. This is much more likely in densely industrial parts of the country. This is where trans-programmatic multimedia models for multi-source chemical transport are most needed.

3.6 Synopsis of Experiences

As one can readily note, there is a very broad range of problems motivating the use and development of risk-based multimedia decision support, modeling, and assessment tools. This range of problems expands the view of multimedia analysis to include problems ranging from contaminant exposure and response to habitat restoration to TMDLs. A common theme of these problems, however, is that they require a more holistic view of problem solving (e.g., linked analysis of watersheds, receiving water, groundwater, and the atmosphere with numerous ecological and human receptors) than is currently the state of practice.

From the information presented above, it is clear that there is a wealth of modeling and analysis tools already being employed across the United States (and by extension, the world) for a very broad range of problems. A cross-section of these tools is presented in the next chapter. Yet, these tools have only limited linkage among themselves and with socio-economic assessment and decision-support tools. Further, these tools lack the full interoperability needed to support the broad spectrum of risk management/decision making required by differing organizations. Thus, while there is great potential for these technologies to help land and water resource managers, they currently are disconnected pieces that need to be blended together into an integrated framework to achieve their highest productivity. Such an integrated framework would need to be designed in an interoperable and extensible fashion that facilitates future technology advancements as well.

4.0 Integrated Multimedia Models and Systems Presented at the Workshop

Prepared by J.W. Buck, T. Nicholson, and G. Whelan

Before discussing and developing key attributes for integrating multimedia models and systems, it is important to gain an understanding of the models and systems currently being used. Background information on integrated multimedia models and systems will help to provide a roadmap for discussing attributes for future models and systems. The specific multimedia models and systems, which were described within this context of the workshop, are presented in this section. It should be noted that a limited number of models and systems was presented, which are considered representative of the models and systems presently used. Inclusion in or absence of multimedia models and systems from the workshop should not constitute endorsement of or objection to other multimedia models and systems.

This chapter is divided by Federal/State Agency (EPA, DOE, NRC, DoD, and State) with each section representing an agency and some of their associated integrated multimedia models and systems. The purpose, general attributes, descriptive summary, selected applications, and summary of each integrated multimedia model and system are discussed.

4.1 DoD's Integrated Multimedia Models and Systems

4.1.1 Army Risk Assessment Management System

4.1.1.1 Purpose and General Attributes of ARAMS

The DoD and the Army use risk-assessment procedures to determine safe levels and cleanup target levels for military-relevant compounds (MRCs) and to evaluate remediation alternatives to provide the most cost-effective approach to reach target levels. As part of the Army's Installation Restoration Research Program (IRRP), ERDC is developing a computer-based, modeling- and database-driven analysis system for estimating human and ecological health impacts and risks associated with MRCs. ARAMS is based on the widely accepted risk paradigm where exposure and effects assessments are integrated to characterize risk. Requirements for ARAMS are shown in Table 4.1.

4.1.1.2 Descriptive Summary of ARAMS

ARAMS is being developed by incorporating various existing databases and models for exposure, intake/uptake, and effects (health impacts) into a conceptual site-modeling framework such that the user has the flexibility to visually specify, through objects, the multimedia pathways and risk scenarios. Also, the user can choose which particular model or database to use for each object. Thus, the hub of ARAMS is the object-oriented CSM. The CSM is based on FRAMES, developed by DOE's PNNL in cooperation with EPA.

Table 4.1. ARAMS Requirements

User and System Requirements	
User Requirements	**System Requirements**
Address MRCs	Provide network-empowered heterogeneous computing
Integrate exposure and effects models and databases	Provide standards for seamless model and data linkages
Provide human and ecological (aquatic and terrestrial) probabilistic risks	Allow integration of legacy models to leverage existing models
Allow screening-level and comprehensive assessments	Provide modularity to add new models/science
Allow multi-level ecological assessments	Provide user interfaces and self-defensive software
Allow for spatially explicit analysis	PC based, Pentium 200 or higher
Provide time-variable analysis (exposure, dose, uptake, effects, risk)	Operates with Windows NT or 2000
Allow multimedia pathways	Can access web-based, network services and remote data
Includes uncertainty analysis	Provide security for military-sensitive issues
Provide linkages to other tools and databases	
Provide user flexibility, such as using measured data and starting anywhere in assessment process	

Before the ARAMS effort, FRAMES handled only human-health assessment, but an ecological health-assessment module has been added through the ARAMS project. A number of other modifications are being made to FRAMES to accommodate ARAMS needs, such as to allow the user to start at any point in conducting the risk-assessment analysis, entering measured exposures, providing additional objects/modules, and adding more functionality. When completed, ARAMS will contain the following basic components:

- Object-oriented, graphical, CSM
- Databases for physical-chemical properties, including bioaccumulation characteristics
- Screening-level fate/transport, exposure-assessment models and options for specifying exposures
- Comprehensive fate/transport, exposure-assessment models
- Databases for human and ecological effects (toxicity reference values)
- Comprehensive ecological effects models, for example, meta-population models
- Assessment of human-health impacts
- Assessment of ecological-health impacts
- Uncertainty-analysis engine
- GIS linkages
- Report generator
- Visualization packages

Version 1.0 of ARAMS is planned for an early FY 2002 release date. This version will allow Level I (e.g., simplified or screening-level) baseline risk assessments. Version 2.0 will host more comprehensive risk-assessment approaches. It is envisioned that there will be updates to the system between Version 1 and 2. Features were added to ARAMS/FRAMES during FY 2000 to allow for ecological risk assessments.

4.1.1.3 Selected Applications of ARAMS

Since ARAMS is a new system still under development, there is no history of applications yet. However, since ARAMS is based on FRAMES and is an extension of the FRAMES capabilities, many of the FRAMES applications are similar to those envisioned for ARAMS. ARAMS/FRAMES is targeted for site-specific, baseline risk assessments. The first planned application of ARAMS is for the Massachusetts Military Reservation (MMR). Results from air dispersion/deposition model simulations of future training scenarios will be used to evaluate human-health impacts associated with soil ingestion, inhalation, and dermal-contact exposure routes.

4.1.2 Land Management System

4.1.2.1 Purpose and General Attributes of LMS

Current technologies offer many capabilities to help managers address these difficult demands, such as GIS, remote sensing, landscape process modeling and simulation, group collaborative forums and conferencing, expert systems, multi-dimensional visualization tools, decision-support systems, and web-based data mining tools. Usage of each of these different technologies is rapidly growing throughout the world. The problem for many users, however, is blending these tools together into a coherent and integrated framework to address management challenges.

Development of integrated computational tools in support of water-resources management for the 21st Century holds significant challenges. The proliferation of the Internet, the need for multimedia analyses, and the integration of socio-economic and physically based modeling are but three of these challenges. ERDC, in concert with other Federal, industrial, and academic partners, is developing LMS to meet these challenges. The LMS provides for state-of-the-art hydro-environmental modeling capabilities, connectivity to geographic information and database systems, and seamless access to web-based network servers.

Inter-operability with other DoD management systems is being stressed. Network-based modeling support is being provided within the system. This capability allows access to remote computing platforms (including DoD high performance computing resources), decentralized databases, and collaborative technical support over network services. Further, the LMS leverages commercial off-the-shelf (COTS) software developments, particularly in the areas of web browsers and standardized data protocols (such as the Open Geospatial Database Interchange [OGDI]). Such leveraging facilitates updating and standardization of the LMS as the marketplace advances.

Decision-support capabilities are also being integrated into LMS to facilitate the interpretation and dissemination of modeling and simulation results, data manipulations, etc., in a manner amenable to differing users at differing levels of the land-management process. This capability will include the development of linkages to key DoD business-process systems that are external to LMS and to certain classes of local-user systems (e.g., GIS and databases) that generally exist at user sites.

LMS is being developed to do the following:

- support multiple applications areas

- integrate predictive capabilities (modeling and simulation), data management, GIS, and heuristics into a decision-support framework

- have collaborative functions (such as multi-user viewing of visualized data) to augment multiple-stakeholder use

- support protocols for interoperability so that modeling results from one model (e.g., watershed model) will interact seamlessly with another model or models (for example, receiving water hydrodynamic and water-quality models)

- be scalable both computationally and conceptually

- have the capability to "learn" from previous modeling efforts or observed experiences

- provide an efficient means to evaluate alternatives and propose new ones as part of the decision-making process

- link effectively to business processes of differing, and often highly disparate, users and stakeholders

- provide three-dimensional visualization and animation capabilities.

The first version of the system, LMS2001, is scheduled to be fielded in July 2001. The system is being validated at four demonstration sites.

4.1.2.2 Descriptive Summary of LMS

The LMS is organized into four levels (Figure 4.1), each with a suite of functions and all accessible through a network-empowered user interface from the user's desktop computer. A general description of the capabilities to be delivered within each of these LMS levels over the system's proposed 6-year-development life cycle is provided below.

- **Decision-Support Level** – The decision-support level is the entry point to all LMS services, and in fact, the ultimate product to the user from the LMS is decision-support technology. This technology is provided by integrating advanced modeling simulation, seamless data access, tradeoff analyses conveying risk and costs of activities, and presentation mechanisms in formats understandable to decision makers and stakeholders in a user-configurable manner. Currently, the system is capable of presenting modeling and simulation results, and all the data inputs thereto, in multi-dimensional visualization formats (including animation), through the on-board capabilities of its Modeling and Simulation Level. Tools are under development, however, to (1) allow decision makers to query databases both from the LMS client and remotely through standard web browsers, (2) modify specific inputs to verified models for new executions, (3) link results to external management software, (4) invoke collaborative functions for multiple-user interaction, and (5) directly compare differing modeled alternatives. In addition, this level of the LMS is being designed to allow users to personalize the data and visual looks they want to observe on a routine basis as a component of network-based profiles that "follow" the user anywhere the Internet reaches. The modeling and simulation (M&S) level houses the

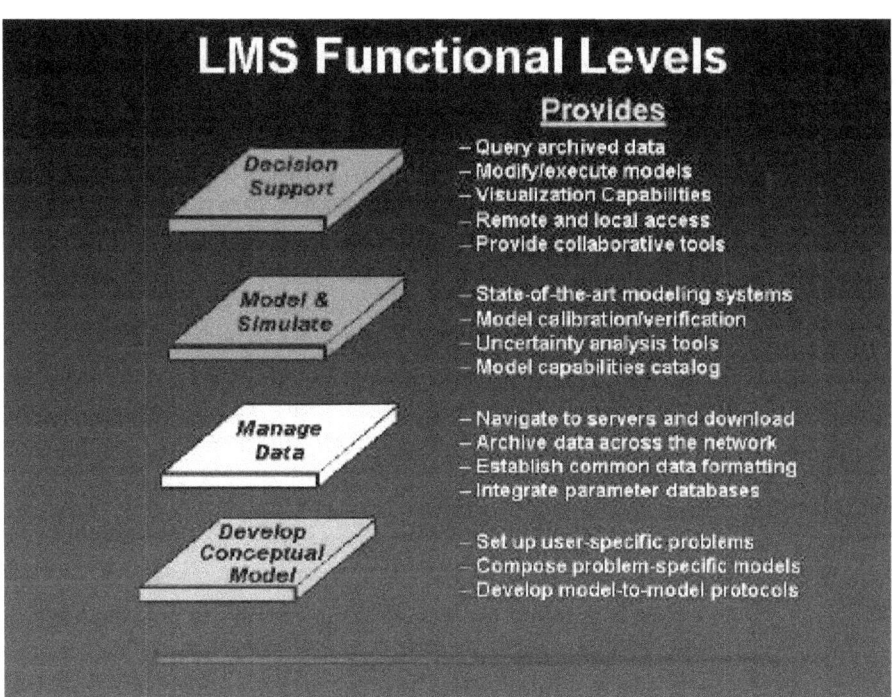

Figure 4.1. LMS Functional Levels

LMS suite of modeling tools, from simple screening tools to highly advanced, three-dimensional models. Protocols and projection methods are being developed to allow M&S results to be interchanged seamlessly between models requiring linkage (e.g., hydrology models and sediment models). Partnering with other agencies is underway to access the best of their existing capabilities without reinventing the wheel. This level provides access to each of the models supported within DoD's Groundwater Modeling System (GMS), Surface Water Modeling System (SMS), and Watershed Modeling System (WMS), respectively, as discussed in more detail at http://chl.wes.army.mil/software. These systems each have state-of-the-art multi-dimensional hydrologic and transport models, visualization, parameterization, and model-conceptualization capabilities. The LMS presently launches each of these three applications. These systems, in concert with the LMS, will also become home to a series of ecological modeling tools. The first capability in this area, a grasslands vegetation model, has been coupled with an overland flow model within the Watershed Modeling System in support of managing military training lands. Note that these coupled models are capable of being executed on a combination of the local client machine and remote computer servers as brokered through the LMS's network services.

- **Modeling and Simulation Level** – The modeling and simulation level includes state-of-the-art modeling systems, model calibration and verification, uncertainty-analysis tools, and a model-capabilities catalog.

- **Manage Data Level** – Among the general design criteria, none is perhaps more important to LMS's productive use than that of being "network-based." The use of the Internet and the world-wide web has become and will continue to be a phenomenon of increasing commercial and social significance. At present, it is common for land managers to require digital elevation

4.5

models, contaminant fate and effects data, installation-management information (location of training areas, firing ranges, roads, buildings, storage facilities, fuel depots, etc.), land cover and use data, and soils information. Adding modeling and simulation results will further increase the number of data types and the volume of data that these managers must assimilate. Further complicating this picture is the ever-expanding view of water-resource projects as components of a holistic landscape that reaches far beyond the installation fence line or the high-water mark of the reservoir. The data needed by land managers (including modeling and simulation results, which can be viewed as a data source for this discussion) are seldom resident on a single computer, or even at a single location. For example, digital elevation information may reside at the local installation or project, but these data often stop at the installation or project boundary. Topographic information, land use and cover, and soils data are all resident through connectivity to network servers throughout the world. Equally, differing environmental-quality modeling and simulation tools can be executed on a variety of computing resources, ranging from personal computers to workstations to high-performance computing resources, through remote network and dial-up connections. The ability of a highly disparate group of users, from range managers to modelers to senior decision makers, to productively access data from environmental-quality decision-support systems is therefore contingent upon those systems facilitating near-seamless connectivity to remote data sources (or, for that matter, data residing on local-area networks within a single office). Ideally, the user will view cyberspace as nothing more than an extension of his/her local machine through the auspices of LMS. LMS R&D associated with data management is focusing on standardizing data gathering, QC, and manipulation from multiple sources (including network-server locations, remotely sensed data, and real-time data, such as weather radar). Parameter databases for the M&S suite will be developed. Standards for model metadata, data interchange between databases and GIS, and linkages to remotely sensed and real-time data will be used as available (e.g., the Tri-Services computer aided drafting design [CADD]/GIS standards) or will be proposed as needed. Several standard functions will be resident on this level. These include fetching data from standardized web-based databases, navigation across networks to user-defined data sources, uploads, downloads, archival, and other activities.

- **Conceptual Model Development Level** – There are two distinct, but interwoven, aspects of conceptualizing a resource problem. The first involves multiple stakeholder development of the resource problem context. In this mode, stakeholders specify their differing priorities for resource allocation, identify key drivers affecting said allocation, and parameterize the constraints associated with differing potential management decisions. The second aspect of conceptualization builds off of, or operates in concert with, the first. This aspect involves the establishment of hypotheses governing the key media (surface water, groundwater, atmosphere, overland flow, etc.) influencing the problem, and the interconnections there between. Note that both aspects of conceptualization are central to (and, in fact often govern) decision making. LMS components are under development to tackle both aspects of conceptualization. Object-oriented developments, such as FRAMES; (http://mepas.pnl.gov:2080/earth/earth.htm) and the DIAS (refer to http://www.dis.anl.gov/DEEM/DIAS) are being evaluated as possible environments to support LMS problem conceptualization. The map-module capabilities of the GMS, SMS, and WMS are being employed as a follow-on means of model conceptualization and setup. Research will continue on these capabilities for at least 2 additional years.

The most basic aspect of LMS is its design as a network-based system. As shown in Figure 4.2, the LMS is designed as a logically three-tiered system with transparent (to the user) connections between the user's local machine, LMS servers, and networked computing and data sources (so-called "back end" computers). This computational design allows for LMS to be operated as either a "thin-client" machine (e.g., use of LMS services through a web browser) or as a "fat-client" machine (e.g., one using a combination of local machine applications and network services). To make the LMS user environment and the LMS cyberspace effective, efficient, and expandable, some general design goals have been adopted for the LMS technology. Note that these are goals for fundamental capabilities to be provided by the underlying framework rather than specific functional goals.

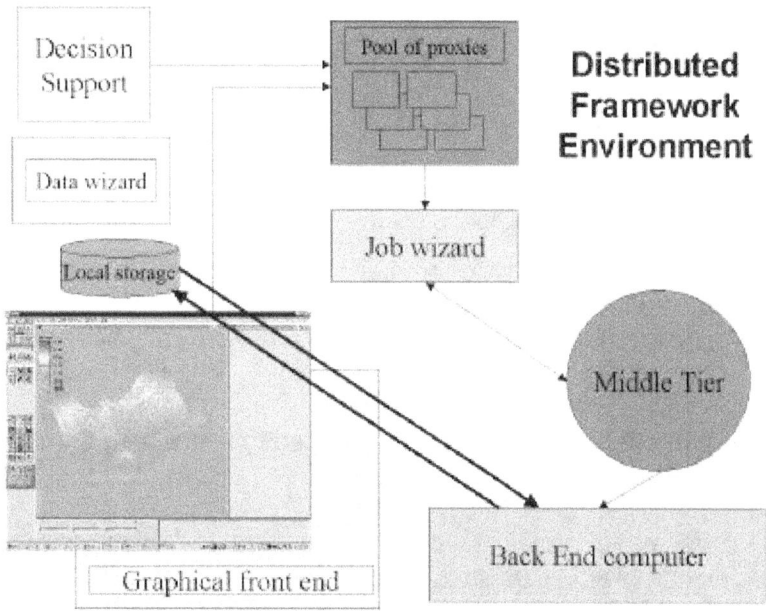

Figure 4.2. LMS Architectural Design

- LMS framework software will be designed for "evolutionary flexibility"; e.g., it will be designed to accommodate change and expansion throughout its life cycle. This is accomplished by using good, professional software engineering practices for all LMS development. Object-oriented methods and tools are the standard.

- LMS will provide seamless access, via a user-friendly graphical user interface (GUI), to a rich set of local and distributed resources (models, data, computers), without requiring the user to gain knowledge of using each resource's host environment (operating system, server software, database management system, etc.) or even to know the location of some resources.

- The LMS environment will accommodate multiple hosts for any type of resource and will provide either automatic or user-selection of the host (e.g., the user may select a host computer to run a tool, or LMS will select one for him/her).

- LMS will provide the ability to readily incorporate legacy models, running locally or remotely, without tailoring the legacy software to the LMS environment. In fact, there will be the capability to allow the user to add legacy software to his/her personal configuration of LMS tools.

- LMS will support interoperable tools using various protocols (which are being defined presently) with inter-operations ranging from simple no-feedback file passing to sophisticated, dynamically interoperable, distributed object-oriented models having significant model-to-model feedback.

- There will be an LMS facility for a user to archive, and readily retrieve, user-selected data and tool output.

- LMS will incorporate security mechanisms and protocols to allow access to security-controlled resources when necessary.

- The LMS client software (e.g., user environment) will have a single, consistent look-and-feel on personal computers running Windows NT/2000 (and subsequent evolutionary operating system [OS]) and on UNIX workstations.

- Vendor-neutral industry standards and commercial software will be used to the greatest extent feasible.

- There will be the facility for automatic distribution of updates to models and data resources.

- Finally, LMS will provide the facility for a user to gain access to all the resources provided without installing any software on his/her local machine other than a standard web browser. This purely web-enabled mode of operation will be a dynamically selectable alternative to the "fat-client" mode.

Some common industry technologies have been adopted to serve as a foundation for building an LMS that achieves these design goals.

- The LMS user interface and framework is built using Java and related technologies. The LMS client, e.g., is a Java program. Design is accomplished using the Unified Modeling Language (UML). However, the LMS development of the LMS client as Win32 rather than pure Java is being assessed presently.

- The LMS will use a common database-management system (presently Oracle), and standard interchanges with existing databases and GIS (through OGDI and Open Geodata Interoperability Standards [OGIS]).

- The Common Object Request Broker Architecture (CORBA) has been adopted (tentatively at this writing) for communication between distributed LMS objects.

- Kerberos Version 5 will be used as the security mechanism for authenticating access to secure resources.

- Microsoft's Windows Terminal Server and Citrix' MetaFrame will be used to provide the browser-only client with the full capabilities of LMS resources hosted in a Windows environment.

4.1.2.3 Selected Applications of LMS

Even though the LMS is a new development, it is being applied at four demonstration sites. These sites include (1) sediment management and land use evaluation in the Redwood Basin of the Minnesota River, (2) permitting and erosion control at 29 Palms Marine Corps base in California, (3) restoration of Peoria Lake, Illinois, and (4) range ecosystem management at Ft. Hood, Texas. In each of these demonstration/application cases, LMS is being used to query data sources over the web, format and input data to watershed and surface-water modeling tools, make predictions regarding likely future outcomes of DoD activities on these watersheds, and present data in ways meaningful to disparate groups over the Internet. These demonstrations and applications are ongoing and will continue throughout 2000 and 2001.

It should be noted that the technology base being employed for predicting the likely outcomes of management decisions on these watersheds involves the use of the Watershed Modeling System and the Surface Water Modeling System (see http://chl.wes.army.mil/software for details on these systems). Thus, while LMS has limited applications, the basic modeling systems underlying LMS's predictive capabilities have had hundreds of applications both nationally and internationally.

4.2 DOE's Integrated Multimedia Models and Systems

Since 1984, DOE has been evaluating, developing, and applying integrated systems software to installation- and complex-wide problems. In addition, the tools that are developed by and for DOE have been applied at SUPERFUND sites and are currently used at a number of universities as part of the teaching curriculum. Since 1977, DOE researchers have been involved in developing and applying numerous physics-based, multimedia models and approaches, including the following:

- DIAS is under development and hopes to represent an object-oriented framework with capabilities for attacking complex modeling and simulation problems. The design of the flexible DIAS software infrastructure will (1) offer the capability to address a complex problem by allowing many disparate multidisciplinary simulation models and other applications to work together within a common framework, (2) integrate existing legacy models, (3) encourage the development of object libraries that contain a large number of reusable objects to represent a wide variety of real-world elements, and (4) operate in a distributed environment where applications can be linked across multiple machines via computer networks. The use and application of DIAS is currently not feasible in its unpackaged state.

- FRAMES (see Section 4.2.1.2 for a descriptive summary of FRAMES).

- GENeration II (Napier et al. 1988) – The GENII computer code was developed at PNNL to incorporate the internal dosimetry models recommended by the International Commission on Radiological Protection (ICRP) into updated versions of existing models for analyzing environmental pathways. The resulting second generation of environmental dosimetry computer codes is compiled in the Hanford Environmental Dosimetry System. The GENII system was developed to provide a state-of-the-art, technically peer-reviewed, documented set of programs for calculating radiation doses from radionuclides released to the environment. Although the codes were developed for use at Hanford, they were designed with the flexibility to accommodate input parameters for a wide variety of generic sites.

- Modular Risk Approach (MRA, started in 1994) (Whelan et al. 1996) – MRA represents an approach that is used to integrate the impacts of multiple waste sites, constituents, environmental settings, environmental media, and exposure routes, loosely coupled to GIS capabilities, on an installation-wide scale.

- RESidual RADioactivity (RESRAD, started in 1991) (Yu et al. 1993) – RESRAD is a set of software codes developed to a multimedia environment, simulating the release, transport, exposures, and health impacts of chemical and radioactive wastes.

- Remediation Options (ReOpt, started in 1989) (Hyman and Bagaasen 1997; PNL 1995) – ReOpt is software that provides suggestions for remedial cleanup alternatives as it functions as an electronic encyclopedia that can be used to sort through environmental remediation processes and their applications.

- Remedial Action Assessment System (RAAS, started in 1987) (Hyman and Bagaasen 1997; PNNL 1996; Hartz and Whelan 1988) – RAAS is a fully coupled remedial-assessment package that investigates remedial alternatives associated with waste-site cleanup and risk reduction associated with the cleanup by providing a comprehensive tool kit for analyzing and evaluating tradeoffs necessary to select a preferred approach for restoring a contaminated site.

- Multimedia Environmental Pollutant Assessment System (MEPAS, started in 1986) (Whelan et al. 1992) – MEPAS sequentially links analytically, semianalytically, and empirically based models to address the release, migration, fate, exposure, and impacts to chemicals and radionuclides at past-practice and active waste sites.

- Remedial Action Priority System (RAPS, started in 1984) (Whelan et al. 1987,1986) – RAPS sequentially linked analytically, semianalytically, and empirically based models to address the release, migration, fate, exposure, and impacts to chemicals and radionuclides at past-practice waste sites.

- Multimedia Contaminant Environmental Exposure Assessment (MCEEA, started in 1982) approach (Onishi et al. 1982) – MCEEA sequentially arranged models, which remained uncoupled, to address typical environmental problems associated with the utility industry

- Chemical Migration and Risk Assessment (CMRA, started in 1977) methodology (Onishi et al. 1985) – CMRA sequentially arranged individual detailed numerical models, which remained uncoupled, to address contaminant migration and fate from agricultural watersheds.

This section provides a more in-depth summary of the applications of the DOE multimedia models and systems presented at the March 2000 Modeling Workshop, including FRAMES and GoldSim. The summary of DOE applications provides insight on how these multimedia models and systems can be used. Although the RESRAD model from ANL was presented at the March 2000 Workshop, the information was not received before the publication of this document. When and if this document is updated, any material from ANL on the RESRAD model will be included.

4.2.1 Framework for Risk Analysis in Multimedia Environmental Systems

4.2.1.1 Purpose and General Attributes of FRAMES

FRAMES was developed by PNNL for DOE's EM, and EPA's ORIA. The original intended function of FRAMES (Version 1.0) was to integrate two multimedia environmental modeling systems (MEPAS from DOE and MMSOILS from EPA) under one framework (Whelan et al. 1998a; 1998b; 1997). This effort proved that similar model types, developed by different agencies, could be integrated under one system and operate as a "new" combination of models with minimum changes to the component legacy codes.

The DOE and EPA have continued to support the development of FRAMES to meet the growing multimedia modeling needs of the Federal agencies. FRAMES has been used on several key DOE applications. The FRAMES concept has also been used by the EPA to develop a nationwide regulatory software system. DoD's USACEs are using FRAMES to support ARAMS. NRC has supported the training of NRC, EPA, DOE, DoD, and Agreement State regulatory staff on the concept of FRAMES and its applications. These training sessions have led to the formation of an active group of developers, some of whom attended and participated in this workshop as described in this document.

See Section 4.2.1.2 for a descriptive summary of FRAMES. FRAMES contains "sockets" for a collection of computer codes that will simulate elements of transport, exposure, and risk assessment, including contaminant source and release to and through overland soils, groundwater in the unsaturated and saturated zones, air, and surface water. FRAMES can simulate exposure assessments for a variety of food-supply scenarios, related receptors, and intake human-health impacts. FRAMES can also assess sensitivity/uncertainty, ecological impacts, and conceptual site design. The "Multimedia" in FRAMES refers to multiple environmental transport pathways and exposure media.

FRAMES has four key functions: (1) facilitate linkage of models under one integrated system using predefined datafile specifications, (2) assist users in defining the conceptual site model using "physical world" module icons, (3) conduct sensitivity and uncertainty analyses on any model integrated, and (4) provide users with graphical and text viewers for analyses of results. Table 4.2 briefly lists the current attributes of the FRAMES software (Version 1.2).

4.2.1.2 Descriptive Summary of FRAMES

Since 1984, PNNL has been developing and applying integrated systems software to DOE site-specific, installation-wide, and complex-wide problems. In addition, the tools that were developed by and for DOE have been applied at SUPERFUND sites and are currently being used at a number of universities as part of the teaching curriculum.

FRAMES (started in 1995) (Whelan et al. 1998a, 1998b, 1997) is an open-architecture, object-oriented framework for assessing hazardous waste sites. It supplies an environmental chemical database, helps the user construct a Conceptual Site Model that is real-world based, allows the user to choose the most appropriate models to solve simulation requirements, and

Table 4.2. List of Attributes of the FRAMES Software Platform

Attribute Number	Attribute Description
1	Operates on IBM-compatible personal computer with at least Windows 95™ or NT
2	Allows the user to integrate new or legacy models using predefined datafile specifications with as few changes to the original codes as possible
3	Allows the user to select the set of modules to define the conceptual site model
4	Allows users to select the contaminants of concern for the modeling scenario, including inorganic, organic, and radionuclides
5	Allows users to conduct sensitivity and uncertainty analyses on developed scenarios; uses any and all models fully integrated and their associated input parameters
6	Allows users to graphically and texturally view the FRAMES predefined datafile specifications
7	Extendable to non-environmental module types, such as cost, remediation, and decision analyses
8	Allows web-based access to models and databases not on the "host" computer
9	Does not "care" what computer language the models are written in
10	Allows for models with different spatial resolutions to be used together
11	Provides online help for FRAMES operation
12	Equal responsibility between the "provider" (e.g., source model) and "consumer" (e.g., unsaturated zone model) module developers for establishing datafile specifications
13	User Manual (Whelan et al. 1997) and online help (linkage within FRAMES to user)

presents graphical packages for analyzing results. FRAMES (1) provides a forum from which various models can interact with each other and (2) facilitates a "plug-and-play" atmosphere to site assessments so modelers can incorporate their own models into the framework to communicate with other assessment software that was previously not available to them.

FRAMES currently includes the MEPAS, GENII-2, and components of the RAAS multimedia models. FRAMES contains sockets for a collection of computer models that simulate elements of a source, fate and transport, exposure, and risk-assessment system. Figure 4.3 provides a diagram of the FRAMES software and the module types currently associated with it. FRAMES has four unique attributes: (1) user friendly, (2) flexible, (3) comprehensive, and 4) application-orientated.

1. **User-Friendly** – FRAMES provides the capability to conceptualize environmental issues using an intuitive drag-and-drop system of icons to construct a pictorial display. Figure 4.3 shows a typical display of a conceptualized environmental issue being modeled in FRAMES. FRAMES employs user-friendly interfaces for easy data entry and model selection. All of FRAMES user interfaces have online help associated with them to provide users with information at their fingertips.

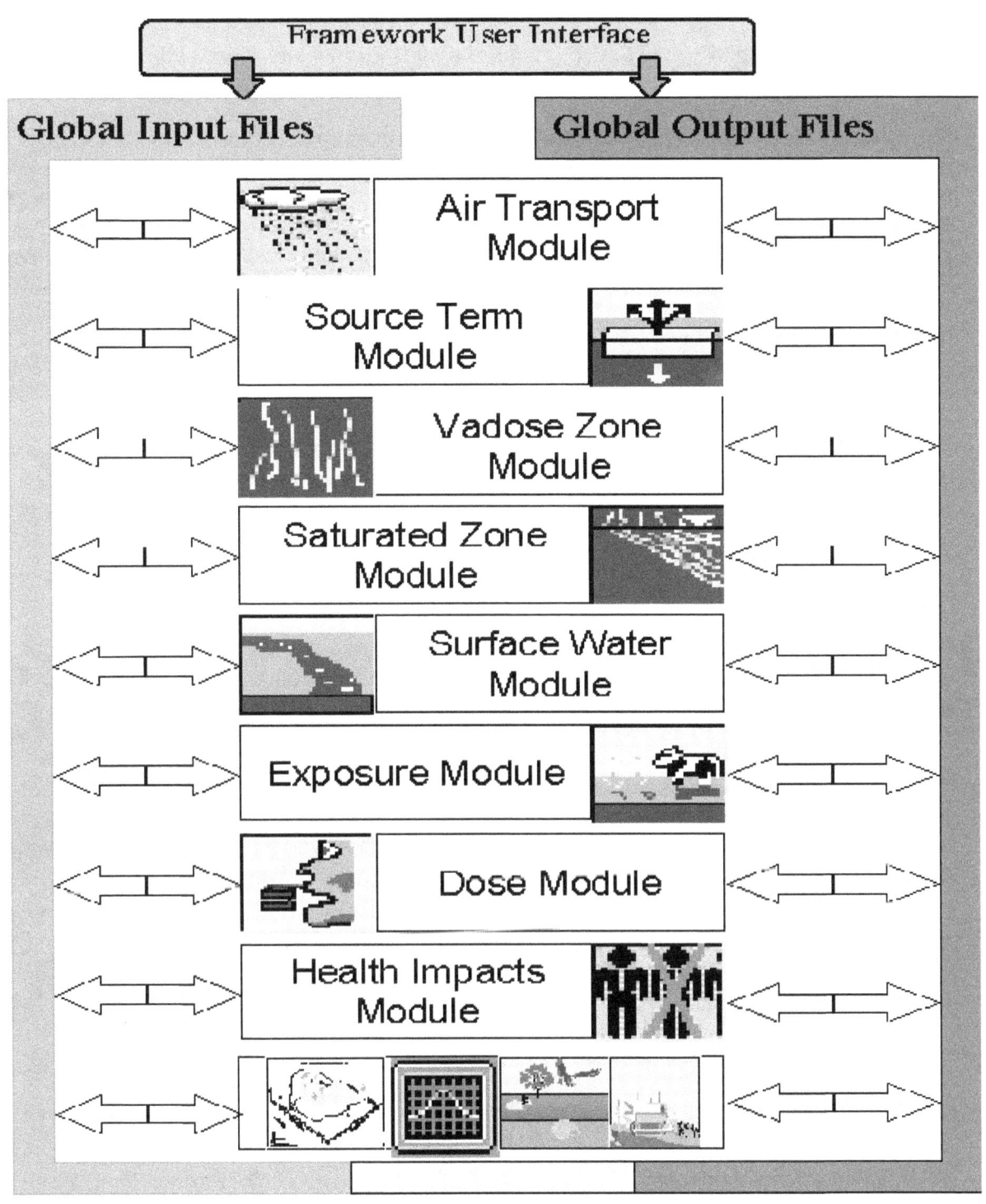

Figure 4.3. Illustrative Linkages Between the Framework User Interface, Global Input/Output Data Files, and Modules in FRAMES

2. **Flexibility** – FRAMES is designed to allow independently developed codes to be fully integrated under it. FRAMES can accommodate codes written in different programming languages. Once a code is fully integrated into FRAMES, it functions with the other integrated codes and FRAMES sensitivity-uncertainty module. With FRAMES, users can develop a personalized modeling system with preferred and/or required codes.

3. **Comprehensive** – FRAMES allows the user to model contaminant movement from its original source, through the environment, and to the environment or human receptors. It also provides their associated health impacts. This type of holistic approach is critical in assessing highly interactive and interrelated issues associated with Environment, Safety, and Health risks. FRAMES allows the user to view modeling information through text, table, and graphical views to confirm and verify the information. In addition, FRAMES provides a method to determine which modeling parameters impact the results the most and the levels of uncertainty involved in the results based on these parameters. This analysis gives managers the critical piece of information missing in many such assessments: What can be changed to lessen environmental impacts? FRAMES is a fully documented software platform and has been co-funded by DOE, EPA, DoD, and Battelle.

4. **Application-Orientated** – This software platform was developed with problem solving in mind and is application-orientated. It combines the best of both government and industrial technical knowledge and expertise. It has been independently reviewed for technical reliability and usability.

4.2.1.3 Selected Applications of FRAMES

FRAMES, and the multimedia models integrated in it, have been used for DOE and other agency applications. FRAMES flexibility allows for a wide range of applications, including site-specific, installation-wide, and nation-wide applications. The following are examples of FRAMES wide range of applications. Site-Specific assessment of FRAMES includes

- Since 1998, FRAMES has been used for the Baseline Risk Assessment at the DOE Pantex Plant in Texas. As a follow-on analysis in 2000, a site-specific evaluation of a waste site was conducted using FRAMES and MEPAS. Detailed source, vadose zone and groundwater modeling was conducted to determine the impact from a perched aquifer.

- FRAMES has been applied at several DoD sites that have been contaminated with an assortment of chemicals. FRAMES allowed DOE and contractors to link their suite of environmental codes with client-preferred codes to provide the appropriate modeling system for the specific application.

Installation-Wide assessments have included the following:

- DOE's TWRS, which evaluated and integrated the impacts, associated 237 tanks containing 177 million curies in 212 million liters to an 80-km radius (DOE 1996).

- FRAMES has been used for the Baseline Risk Assessment at the DOE Pantex Plant (1998) in Texas. A site-specific groundwater transport code was linked into FRAMES and its models to conduct a source-to-impacts analysis. Multiple waste sites were evaluated for the assessment to estimate the human and ecological impacts from the Pantex Plant.

PNNL conducted a nationwide assessment of FRAMES for the EPA. The FRAMES concept and datafile specifications were critical components of EPA's HWIR. FRAMES concepts were used to integrate selected fate, transport, exposure, and impact codes to develop nationwide regulatory information. PNNL received the highest technical and management marks possible from the EPA client.

4.2.2 GoldSim System

4.2.2.1 Purpose and General Attributes of GoldSim

GoldSim is a proprietary powerful and flexible Windows-based computer program for carrying out probabilistic simulations of complex systems to support management and decision-making in engineering, science, and business (Kossik and Miller 2001a,b). The program, developed by Golder Associates Inc., is highly-graphical, highly extensible, capable of directly representing uncertainty, and allows you to create compelling presentations of your model. Although GoldSim can be used to solve a wide variety of complex problems, it is particularly well-suited (and was originally developed) to support an evaluation of existing and proposed radioactive-waste-management facilities. Powerful contaminant-transport features allow nearly any kind of natural or man-made environmental system to be simulated. The program was developed with funding from Golder Associates, DOE's Yucca Mountain Project, the Japan Nuclear Cycle Development Institute (JNC), and Empresa Nacional de Residuos Radioactivos, S.A. (Enresa). This proprietary program was specifically developed to address three problems that are common to most complex environmental modeling efforts:

- For most real-world applications, a large degree of uncertainty usually exists with regard to the controlling parameters and processes. When carrying out predictive simulations, these uncertainties cannot be properly represented using deterministic techniques alone.

- Most modeling efforts are multi-disciplinary in nature. Unfortunately, in such efforts, it is easy for individuals building sub-models to get caught up in the details of their model and lose sight of the "big picture" (the ultimate problem that the model is trying to address). The end result is typically separate sub-models that are unjustifiably complex. More important, the complex interactions and interdependencies between subsystems are often ignored or poorly represented.

- Many complex environmental models are built such that they can only be understood and explained by the people who developed them. A model that cannot be easily understood (by decision-makers or the public) is a model that will not be used.

Although these problems occur in nearly any kind of complex environmental modeling effort, they are particularly relevant to modeling the performance of proposed and existing radioactive-waste-management facilities (due to the very long time frames involved, the large uncertainties, and the public's reaction to radioactive-waste issues). The result of more than 10 years of development effort, GoldSim was specifically designed to

- explicitly represent uncertainty in processes, parameters, and events

- facilitate a "top-down" total system modeling approach aimed at integrating all aspects of the system and keeping a modeling effort focused on the "big picture"

- facilitate the documentation and presentation of complex models to multiple audiences at an appropriate level.

4.2.2.2 Descriptive Summary of GoldSim

GoldSim is a proprietary powerful and flexible platform for visualizing and numerically simulating nearly any kind of physical, financial, or organizational system. In a sense, GoldSim is like a "visual spreadsheet" that allows you to visually create and manipulate data and equations. Unlike spreadsheets, however, GoldSim allows you to readily evaluate how systems evolve over time and predict their future behavior. Because simulation can be such a powerful tool for understanding and managing complex systems, a variety of simulation tools currently exist. The following combination of features, however, makes the GoldSim approach unique:

- GoldSim is user-friendly and highly graphical, such that you can literally draw (and subsequently present) a picture (an influence diagram) of your system in an intuitive way without having to learn any arcane symbols or notation.

- GoldSim is extremely flexible, allowing it to be applied to nearly any kind of system. The software allows you to build a model of your system in a hierarchical, modular manner, such that the model can readily evolve as more knowledge regarding the system is obtained. Hence, a GoldSim model can be very simple or extremely complex.

- Uncertainty in processes, parameters, and future events can be explicitly represented. Uncertainty in processes and parameters can be represented by specifying model inputs as probability distributions. The impact of uncertain events (e.g., earthquakes, floods, sabotage) can also be directly represented by specifying the occurrence rates and consequences of such "disruptive events."

- GoldSim is highly extensible. You can dynamically link external programs or spreadsheets directly into your GoldSim model. In addition, GoldSim was specifically designed to support the addition of customized modules (program extensions) to address specialized applications.

- GoldSim allows you to create compelling presentations of your model. A model that cannot be easily explained is a model that will not be used or believed. GoldSim was specifically designed to allow you to effectively document, explain, and present your model. You can add graphics, explanatory text, notes and hyperlinks to your model, and organize it in a hierarchical manner such that it can be presented at an appropriate level of detail to multiple target audiences.

These features allow GoldSim to be applied at multiple levels, depending on the nature of the application: powerful, flexible simulator; system integrator; and visual information management system. Figure 4.4 presents an illustrative example of a GoldSim User Interface Application. At the most fundamental level, GoldSim can be used as a powerful, flexible simulator. That is, you may only wish to apply it to a very specific problem addressing one aspect of a complex system (e.g., behavior of an engineered barrier, a site-wide water balance, or movement of contaminants through groundwater or another pathway). The GoldSim simulation environment is highly graphical and completely object-oriented. That is, you create, document, and present models by creating and manipulating graphical objects (referred to as elements) representing data and relationships between the data, as illustrated by Figure 4.5.

In a sense, GoldSim is like a "visual spreadsheet," allowing you to visually create and manipulate data and equations. As can be seen in the simple example shown above, based on how the various objects in your model are related, GoldSim automatically indicates their influences and interdependencies by visually connecting them in an appropriate manner. GoldSim provides a wide variety of built-in objects from which you can construct your models, and, if desired, you can program your own custom objects and link them seamlessly into the GoldSim framework. In addition, GoldSim can dynamically link to spreadsheets and user-provided models. For example, it can dynamically transfer data into an Excel spreadsheet, recalculate the spreadsheet, and retrieve results from the spreadsheet and propagate them to the rest of the GoldSim model. Where user-provided models are integrated with GoldSim, it is necessary to convert them into a subroutine within a DLL library, which GoldSim calls at each time step with updated input data. The conversion process can be fairly straightforward or relatively complex, depending on the structure of the user-provided model. GoldSim's graphical interface and powerful computational features facilitate a wide range of simulations, ranging from a simple screening analysis assignment put together in less than an hour to a complex application built over a period of several months. Because GoldSim is flexible and powerful enough to represent practically any aspect of your system and provides unique capabilities for building your model in a hierarchical, modular manner, it is ideally suited to act as a system integrator: a total system model focused on creating a consistent framework in which all aspects of the system, as well as the complex interactions and interdependencies between subsystems, can be represented. This was the original and primary use for which GoldSim was designed, as illustrated by Figure 4.6.

Complex models often require a great detail of input data. These inputs may reside in databases, spreadsheets, or in written documentation. The user of a model (e.g., the author of the model, a reviewer of the model, or a decision-maker evaluating the results) can be most effective if this input information can be visually integrated with (and readily accessed and viewed alongside) the simulation model. At the highest and most powerful level, GoldSim can be used as a visual information-management system, providing you with the ability to directly link to data sources, as well as describe, document and explain your model in a compelling and effective manner to any audience, as illustrated by Figure 4.7.

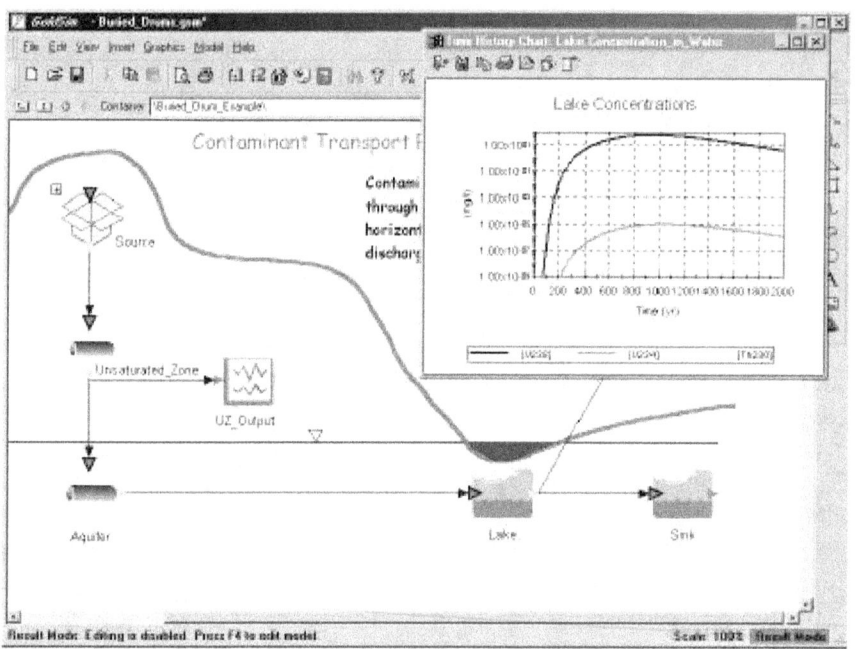

Figure 4.4. Example of a GoldSim User Interface Application

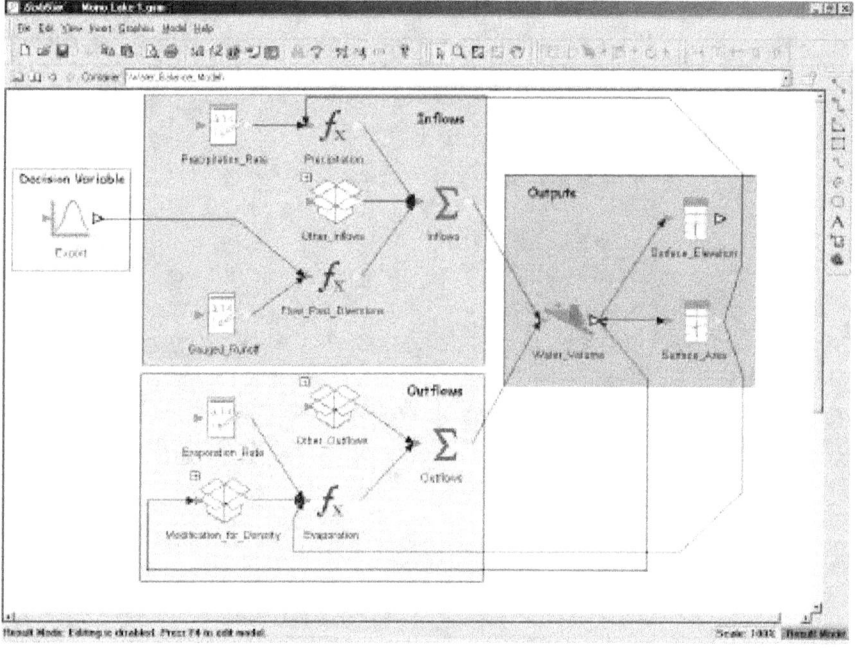

Figure 4.5. Illustrating the Creation and Manipulation of Graphical Objects, Representing Data and Relationships Between Data

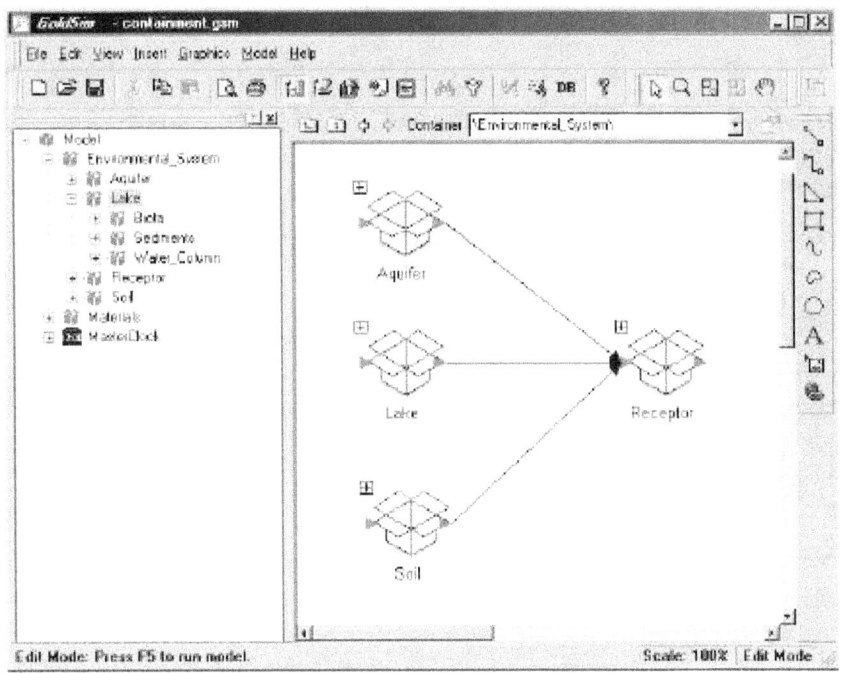

Figure 4.6. Schematic Illustrating the Integration of Sub-Models in GoldSim

The Contaminant Transport Module allows the user to explicitly represent the following processes:

- Release of mass (e.g., contaminants) from specified sources, taking into account both the failure of containers (e.g., drums) in which the contaminants are disposed and the degradation of any materials in which the contaminants are bound (e.g., grout, metal, glass).

- Transport of contaminants through multiple transport pathways within an environmental system (e.g., aquifers, streams, atmosphere). The transport pathways can consist of multiple transport and storage media (e.g., groundwater, surface water, air, soil), and both advective and diffusive transport mechanisms can be directly simulated. Transport processes incorporate solubility constraints and partitioning of contaminants between the media present in the system, and they can include the effects of complex chemical reactions and decay processes. Transport processes occurring within fractured rock (e.g., matrix diffusion) can also be simulated.

- Biological transfer of contaminants within or between organisms. Like physical transport pathways, biological transport pathways can consist of any number of transport and storage media (for example, blood, tissue) that can be linked by a variety of transport mechanisms.

The Contaminant Transport Module provides this special functionality by adding specialized elements for representing contaminant species, transport media, transport pathways, contaminant sources, and receptors to the GoldSim simulation framework, as illustrated by the icons shown in

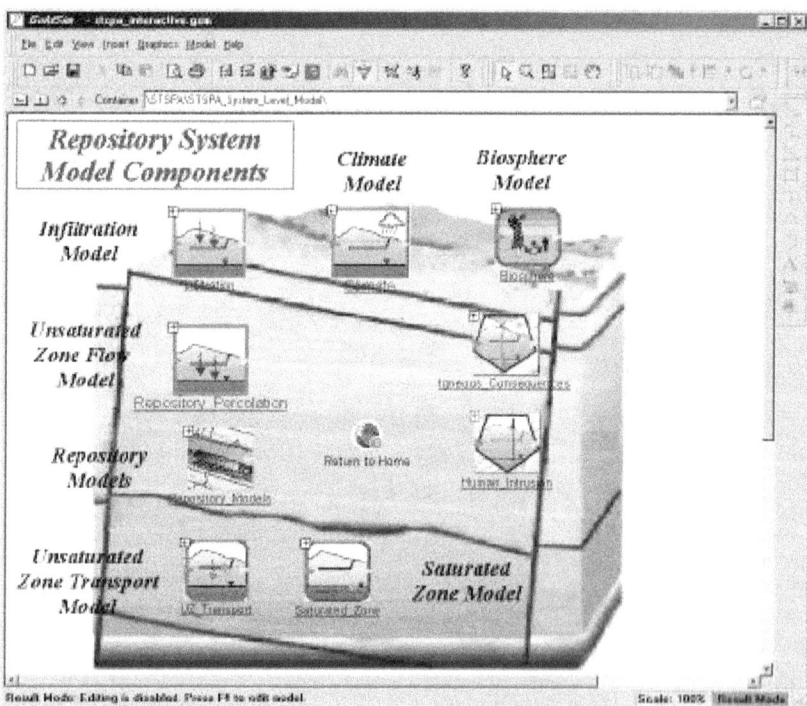

Figure 4.7. Schematic Illustrating the Visual Information Management System of GoldSim

Figure 4.8. By linking these environmental elements together (and integrating them with GoldSim's basic elements), you can build simple and complex contaminant transport simulations, as illustrated in Figure 4.9.

4.2.2.3 Selected Applications of GoldSim

GoldSim was originally developed to assist the DOE in evaluating the potential high-level radioactive waste repository at Yucca Mountain, Nevada. It is currently being used to help design remediation measures for contaminated sites and to evaluate the safety of proposed radioactive waste disposal facilities worldwide. A few of these applications are listed below:

- Evaluation of Potential Yucca Mountain Repository, Nevada. DOE has been using GoldSim (and an earlier version of the software called RIP) to evaluate the safety of the proposed repository for the nation's spent nuclear fuel at Yucca Mountain, Nevada, since 1992. GoldSim is currently being used to support the Site Recommendation to the President, and if approved, will be used to support the License Application for the site.

- International Radioactive Waste Disposal Research. ENRESA, the Spanish radioactive waste-management agency, has been using GoldSim (and RIP) since 1992 to evaluate potential host rocks as part of a program to select a disposal site for the nation's spent nuclear fuel. GoldSim is also being used by the French (ANDRA), Taiwanese (INER), and Japanese (JNC) programs to manage high-level radioactive wastes.

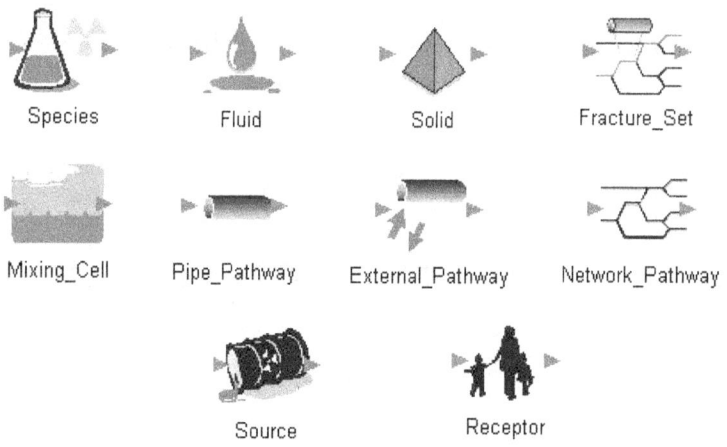

Figure 4.8. Elements for Representing Contaminant Species, Transport Media and Pathways, Contaminant Sources, and Receptors

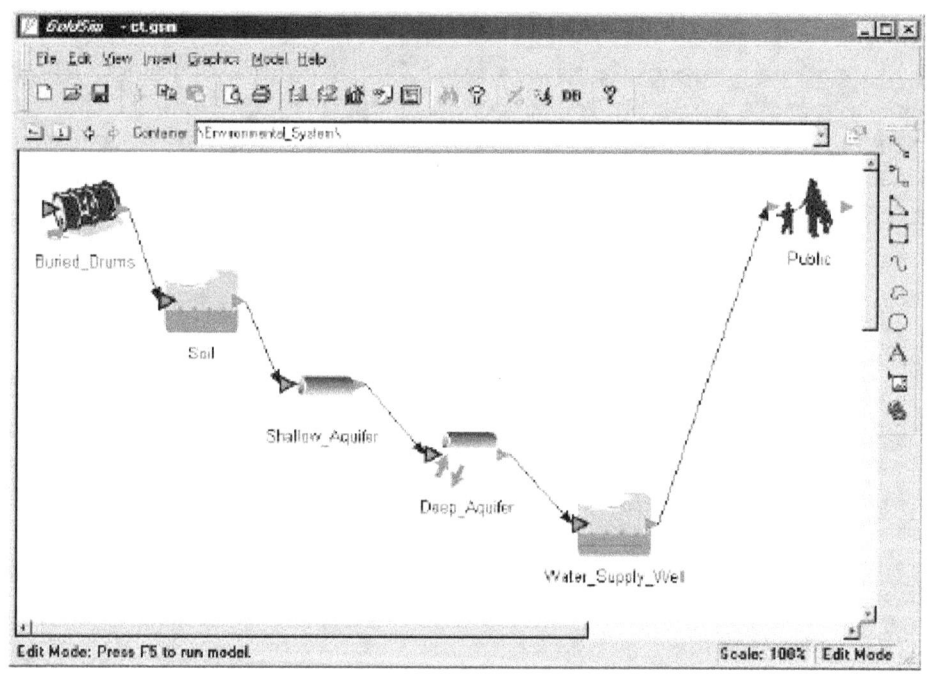

Figure 4.9. Schematic Illustrating a Contaminant Transport Simulation in GoldSim

- Evaluation of Waste Disposal Sites, Los Alamos, New Mexico. Los Alamos National Laboratory is using GoldSim to aid in characterizing risks and to help identify monitoring requirements for areas in which to dispose of low-level radioactive wastes.

- Remediation and Closure of Uranium Mill Tailings and Mine Workings. GoldSim is being used in Germany and Canada to evaluate alternative remediation and closure options for abandoned mine workings and tailings facilities associated with former uranium mining operations.

- Waste Isolation Pilot Plant (WIPP), Carlsbad, New Mexico. DOE has used GoldSim (and RIP) since 1994 at the WIPP site to perform sensitivity calculations for various processes and to supplement performance assessment (PA) efforts being led by Sandia National Laboratories.

- Evaluation of Underground Nuclear Test Sites, Nevada. GoldSim was used to evaluate the influence of different conceptual models of the (highly uncertain) groundwater flow system on estimates of the extent of radionuclide migration from underground nuclear test sites within the Frenchman Flat corrective action unit at the Nevada Test Site.

- Evaluation of Closure and Operational Options for Mines. GoldSim has been used in the United States, Canada, Europe, and Asia to evaluate alternative closure and operational options for existing and proposed mines.

4.3 EPA's Integrated Multimedia Models and Systems

4.3.1 Multimedia, Multi-pathway, Multiple Receptor Risk Assessment

4.3.1.1 Purpose and General Attributes of 3MRA

The 3MRA model is being developed by EPA's OSW and ORD. The goal of the 3MRA model is to provide a risk-assessment modeling tool for OSW to support regulatory and management decisions under RCRA. The model estimates exemption levels below which chemicals in wastes currently identified as Subtitle C hazardous waste could be disposed of in nonhazardous waste-management units. These standards would protect the health of humans and other living organisms, yet allow the waste to exit the hazardous-waste category under RCRA, Subtitle C. To set national criteria, EPA sponsored the development and implementation of the 3MRA, which consists of a system user interface, 5 databases, 17 modules (5 source terms, 5 fate and transport, 3 food chains, 2 exposure [human and ecological], 2 risk/hazard [human and ecological]), and 6 data processors. The software system accounts for organic and inorganic chemicals, geographic setting, and distance from a waste site. For human-health analyses, the system accounts for exposure pathway (e.g., inhalation and ingestion), receptor types (e.g., resident, fisher, and farmer), and age groups. For ecological analyses, the system accounts for habitat and receptor groups (e.g., aquatic and bird, respectively), habitat types (e.g., grassland), and trophic levels (e.g., producers). The following general attributes are part of the 3MRA model:

- designed with object-oriented programming, allowing for easy connectivity or replacement of modules through predefined data specifications

- operates on IBM compatible personal computer with at least Windows 95™

- accommodates a variety of programming languages for the modules

- has a user interface, although minimal information is expected from the user

- allows assessment of risks across several environmental media and exposure pathways for both human and ecological receptors

- produces a variety of output files that allow a user to understand the impacts of a chemical-specific level on various receptor types, age groups, and exposure pathways.

4.3.1.2 Descriptive Summary of 3MRA

The 3MRA model is an integrated, multimedia, multi-pathway, and multiple receptor risk-assessment system that evaluates impacts to human and ecological receptors at a national scale. The model estimates risks that might occur from the long-term, multimedia release of a chemical from five types of waste management units (landfill, waste pile, land-application unit, surface impoundment, and aerated tank). The model provides flexibility in producing a distribution of risk outputs to describe the range of individual risks across the nation from potential exposures to chemicals in waste. The 3MRA model includes the chemical partitioning, release, fate, exposure, and risk modules, and the input data for the modules (e.g., environmental setting, chemical, and meteorological data). The model contains both legacy models and newly created modules and data sets. The model incorporates interacting modules that include the following:

- source modules that estimate the simultaneous chemical mass losses to the different media and maintain the chemical mass balance of the releases from the waste-management unit into the environment over time

- fate/transport modules that receive calculated releases from waste-management units and distribute the mass through each of the media to determine the chemical concentrations in air, groundwater, soil, and surface water across space and time

- food-chain modules that receive the outputs from the fate and transport modules and estimate the uptake of chemicals in various plants and animals

- exposure modules that use the media concentrations from the fate and transport modules to determine the exposure to human and ecological receptors from inhalation (for humans only), direct contact (for ecological receptors only) and ingestion (for both receptor types)

- risk modules that predict the risk/hazard quotient for each receptor of concern.

The 3MRA system technology was designed to incorporate software modules representing individual steps of a risk assessment (e.g., source release of contaminants, fate and transport in various environmental media, exposure, etc.) within a software framework that manages and processes the information flow through the system. A simple schematic showing the relationships of the various data processors, modules, and databases in the 3MRA are shown in Figure 4.10.

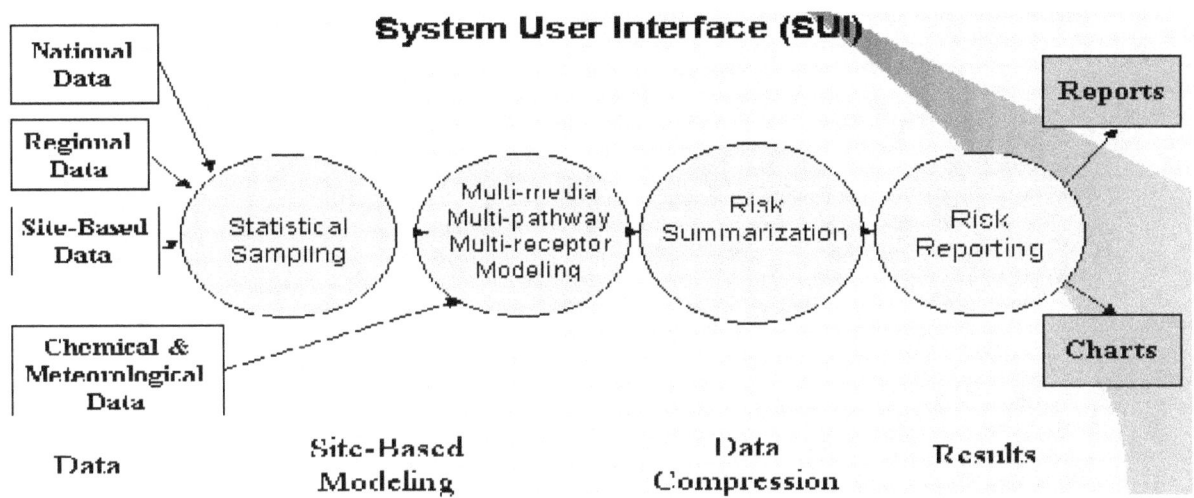

Figure 4.10. Simplified View of 3MRA Software System (After Whelan and Laniak 1998a)

The software framework was designed using "object-oriented design" and, as such, allowed for the decoupling of individual modules. This design greatly improved the ability of module developers (e.g., a modeler developing a new surface water module) to "plug" the new module into a full multimedia modeling system without the need to develop a complete modeling system. The 3MRA was designed to facilitate a national assessment and thus currently does not contain a site-specific user interface.

The model is implemented on a site-by-site basis to generate estimates at the national level. The model assesses risks to human and ecological receptors who might live within 2 km of a waste-management unit. For all locations at each site where there is a receptor, the model calculates the simultaneous exposures and resulting risks for that receptor by adding the appropriate series of pathway-specific risks. Some of the modeled receptors might be exposed through several pathways, some might only be exposed through one pathway, and some might not be exposed at all to any pathway. From this information, the model generates, for each chemical across all sites, a distribution of risk for each receptor type (and also for all receptor types). This distribution of risk is also calculated for each of three radial distances (500 m, 1000 m, and 2000 m) from the center of the waste-management units.

The 3MRA model currently is set up to evaluate risks at 201 sites across the United States. These sites are meant to be representative of sites where potentially exempted hazardous waste may be disposed of. A simplified layout for a site is shown in Figure 4.11 in which human receptors, various types of water bodies, habitats, and farms are located with respect to a waste-management unit present in the center of the 2-km area of interest. The model requires more than 700 input parameters covering a wide range of general data categories, including (1) waste-management unit characteristics, (2) meteorological data, surface water, and watershed characteristics, (3) soil properties, (4) aquifer properties, (5) food-chain or food-web characteristics, (6) human and

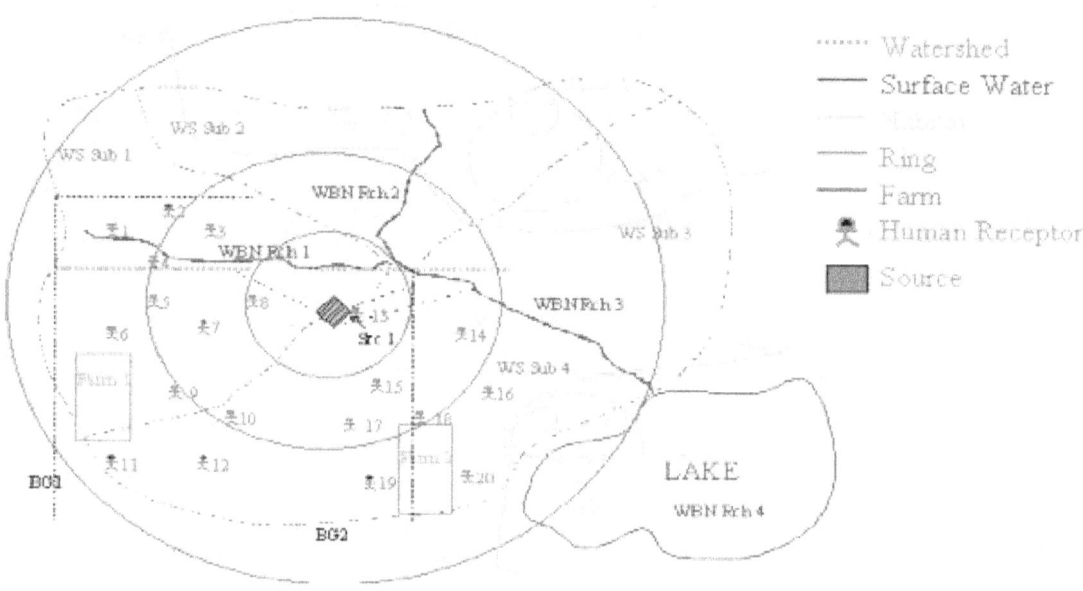

Figure 4.11. Example 3MRA Site Spatial Layout (1/10th Scale)

ecological exposure factors, (7) types and locations of human and ecological receptors and habitats surrounding the waste-management unit, and (8) chemical-specific properties and toxicity values. The model is intended to be implemented on a national scale, but is based on a regional, site-based approach. In this approach, site-based data are used when readily available as inputs to the model. When site-based data are not readily available, parameters are then populated from data collected on a regional level, followed by national-level data. Table 4.3 shows the level of specificity (site-based, regional, national) by data category that have been currently collected for use in the 3MRA.

The 3MRA model and its components are expected to complete external peer review during Summer 2001 and review by EPA's Science Advisory Board in 2002. Comprehensive internal and independent testing of the model has been completed, and Version 1.0 is now available. Modifications to Version 1.0 are currently underway based on comments from the external peer reviewers and the public. The model, data, and documentation are available on the Web at http://www.epa.gov/epaoswer/hazwaste/id/hwirwste/risk.htm.

4.3.1.3 Selected Applications of 3MRA

The 3MRA model has not been formerly applied in a regulatory context. It is intended to be applied in the context of generating exemption levels for low-risk wastes to be eligible for exit from the Subtitle C regulations under RCRA as part of HWIR. With additional modifications underway, additional projects within OSW are expected to use future versions of the model. However, individual modules and data sets from the model have been used in various decision-making projects within OSW.

Table 4.3. Levels of Data Collected for the 3MRA

DATA CATEGORY	SITE-BASED	REGIONAL	NATIONAL
Waste Management Unit	•		•
Waste Properties			•
Meteorological		•	
Watershed and Waterbody Layout	•		
Surface Water		•	•
Soil/vadose Zone	•		•
Aquifer		•	•
Farm Food Chain/Terrestrial Food Web			•
Aquatic Food Web		•	•
Human Exposure Factors			•
Ecological-Exposure Factors		•	•
Chemical Properties			•
Biouptake/Bioaccumulation Factors			•
Human-Health Benchmarks			•
Human-Receptor Type and Location	•		•
Ecological Benchmarks			•
Ecological Receptors	•	•	
Ecological-Habitat Type and Location	•	•	

4.3.2 MODELS-3

4.3.2.1 Purpose and General Attributes of Models-3

Environmental problems are growing in complexity and scope. Local management solutions alone can no longer address many of today's problems. Regional and occasionally even global coordinated efforts are needed. Accordingly, the models we use to assess these problems and evaluate alternative solutions are increasing in complexity. Many researchers, both in the United States and other countries, are engaged in research and model development to help address these environmental problems. But, without sufficient coordination, it will be extremely difficult to integrate these individual efforts into a comprehensive assessment. Thus, the concept of an integrated modeling and analysis framework, Models-3/Community Multiscale Air Quality (CMAQ), was formulated.

With Models-3, it may be possible to begin leveraging upon the scientific and technology advancements of other federal agencies, academia, and research institutions, thereby evolving toward a more unified comprehensive approach to multi-discipline environmental modeling. Because the scope of such a system is extremely large, we limited the initial Models-3 system-development effort to air-quality modeling. Therefore, the primary goals for the Models-3 modeling system are to improve 1) the EM community's ability to evaluate the impact of air-quality management practices for multiple pollutants at multiple scales and 2) the scientist's ability to better probe, understand, and simulate chemical and physical interactions in the atmosphere. These two groups—the model user and the model developer—have very different requirements for a modeling framework. However, there are significant advantages in using the same problem solving environment. Thus, Models-3 is intended to serve as a community foundation for the widespread application of air-quality models and for their continued scientific advancement. Models-3 is not a single model or modeling system, but rather, it is a problem-solving environment containing components that help you build, evaluate, and apply air-quality models.

The initial version of Models-3 contains a CMAQ modeling system for urban- to regional-scale air-quality simulation of tropospheric ozone, acid deposition, visibility, and fine particulate. Models-3 and CMAQ in combination form a powerful third-generation air-quality modeling and assessment system. First-generation air-quality models dealt with tropospheric air quality with simple chemistry at local scales using Gaussian plume formulation as the basis for prediction. Second-generation models covered a broader range of scales (local, urban, regional) and pollutants, addressing each scale with a separate model and often focusing on a single pollutant. Third-generation models treat multiple pollutants simultaneously up to continental scales and incorporate feedbacks between chemical and meteorological components. Future efforts toward fourth-generation systems will extend linkages and process feedback to include air, water, land, and biota to simulate the transport and fate of chemicals and nutrients throughout an ecosystem.

4.3.2.2 Descriptive Summary of Models-3

Models-3 Modeling and Analysis Systems – The Models-3 release contains three types of environmental modeling systems: meteorological, emission, and chemistry transport. It also includes a visualization and analysis system. Figures 4.12 and 4.13 illustrate the relationship between and components within these systems. The purpose of each of these systems and a brief introduction are as follows:

- Meteorological Modeling System – provides descriptions of atmospheric motions; fields of pressure, moisture, and temperature; fluxes of momentum, moisture, and heat; turbulence characteristics; clouds and precipitation; and atmospheric radiative characteristics. The MM5 meteorological modeling system in this Models-3 release contains five individual processors. These processors include the TERRAIN processor for defining the simulation domain, the DATAGRID processor for processing background fields, the RAWINS processor for objective analysis, the INTERP processor for setting the initial and boundary conditions for the meteorological model, and the MM5v2 main-model processor.

- Emission Modeling System – simulates trace gas and particulate emission into the atmosphere, depending on surrounding meteorological conditions and socioeconomic activities. Typically, emissions are broken down into point sources, line sources (on-road mobile), and area sources. A point source tracks emissions from a single source (e.g., a boiler stack or dry cleaner). A line source tracks emissions that follow a road (e.g., cars or trucks). Area sources include off-road mobile sources, biogenic emissions, and other sources that are often related to the earth's surface where humans, animals, and plants reside. The Models-3 Emission Projection and Processing System (MEPPS) in this Models-3 release contains 5 individual processors. These processors include the Inventory Data Analyzer (IDA), Input Emission Processor (INPRO), Emission Processor (EMPRO), Output Processor (OUTPRO), and Models-3 Emission Projections Processor (MEPPRO).

- Chemistry Transport Modeling System – simulates various chemical and physical processes that are thought to be important for understanding atmospheric trace gas transformations and distributions. Generally, the chemistry-transport model relies on a meteorological model to describe atmospheric states and motions and depends on emission models for the anthropogenic and biogenic emissions that are injected into the atmosphere. The chemical transport modeling system in this Models-3 release contains eight individual processors. These processors include a Land-Use Processor (LUPROC), a Meteorology-Chemistry Interface Processor (MCIP), an Emissions-Chemistry Interface Processor (ECIP), Photolysis Rate Processor (JPROC), Initial Conditions Processor (ICON), Boundary Conditions Processor (BCON), Main Chemical-Transport Model Processor (CCTM), and Process Analysis Processor (PROCAN).

- Visualization and Analysis System – plots and graphs data that have been created by one of the Models-3 modeling systems or that have been imported into Models-3. Visualization techniques are an important part of air-quality data analysis. The Models-3 visualization and analysis system provides several packages that can plot or graph data.

Three-dimensional animation capabilities are also provided in the system. The visualization and analysis system in this Models-3 release contains two individual visualization packages.

These packages include Vis5D five-dimensional visualization package (Package for Analysis and Visualization of Environmental Data [PAVE]) application for visualizing multivariate and gridded datasets. The following three commercial visualization and analysis packages function as an integral part of Models-3, but must be acquired and installed separately:

1. DX Driver for launching the IBM Visualization Data Explorer, which can handle some visualizations of which the other packages are not capable, such as multiple/nested and terrain following grids (free download).

2. Statistical Analysis System (SAS®) (Purchase)

3. Arc/Info (Purchase)

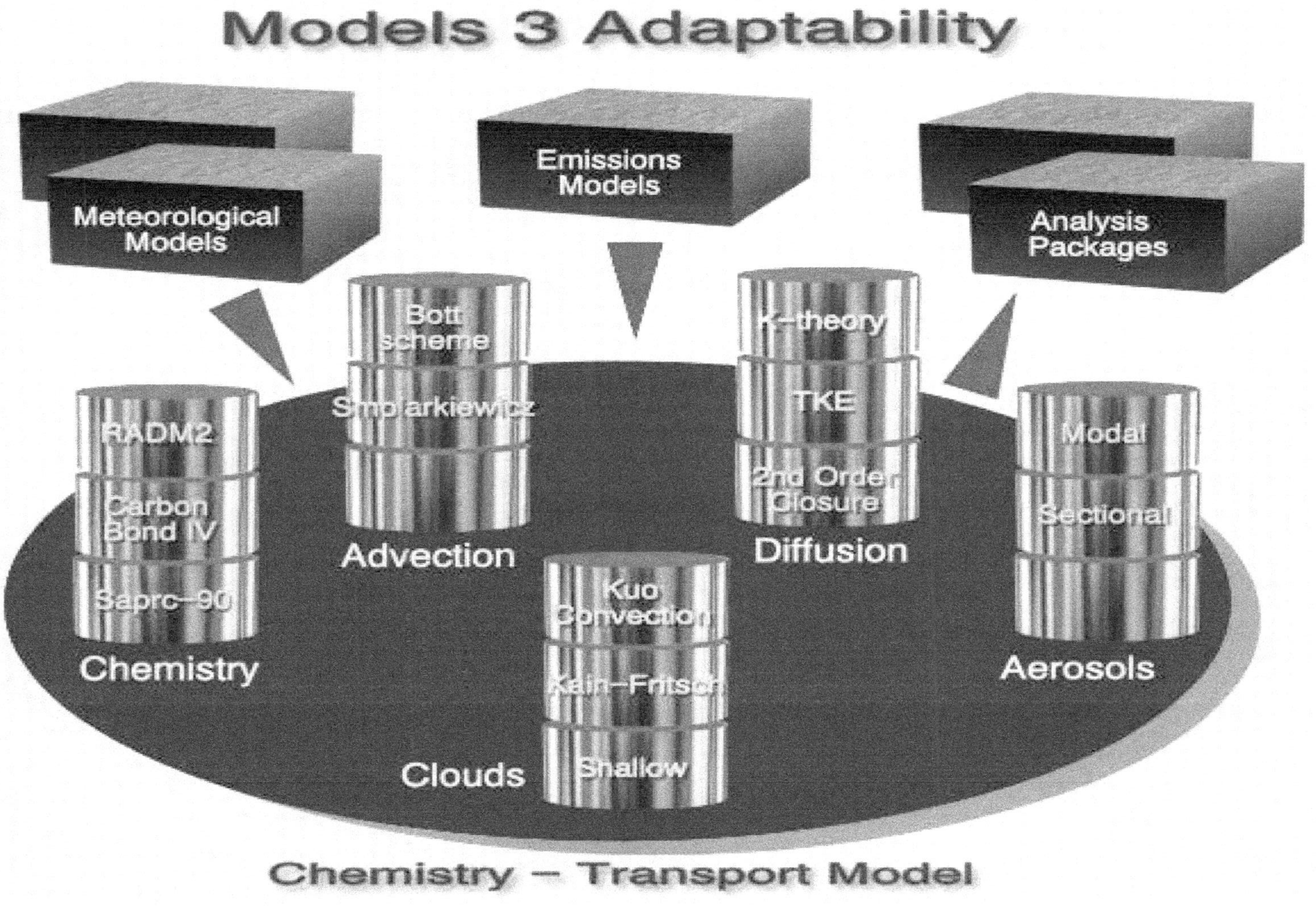

Figure 4.12. Models-3 Relationship Between Meteorological, Emission, and Chemistry Transport Environmental Modeling Systems

4.31

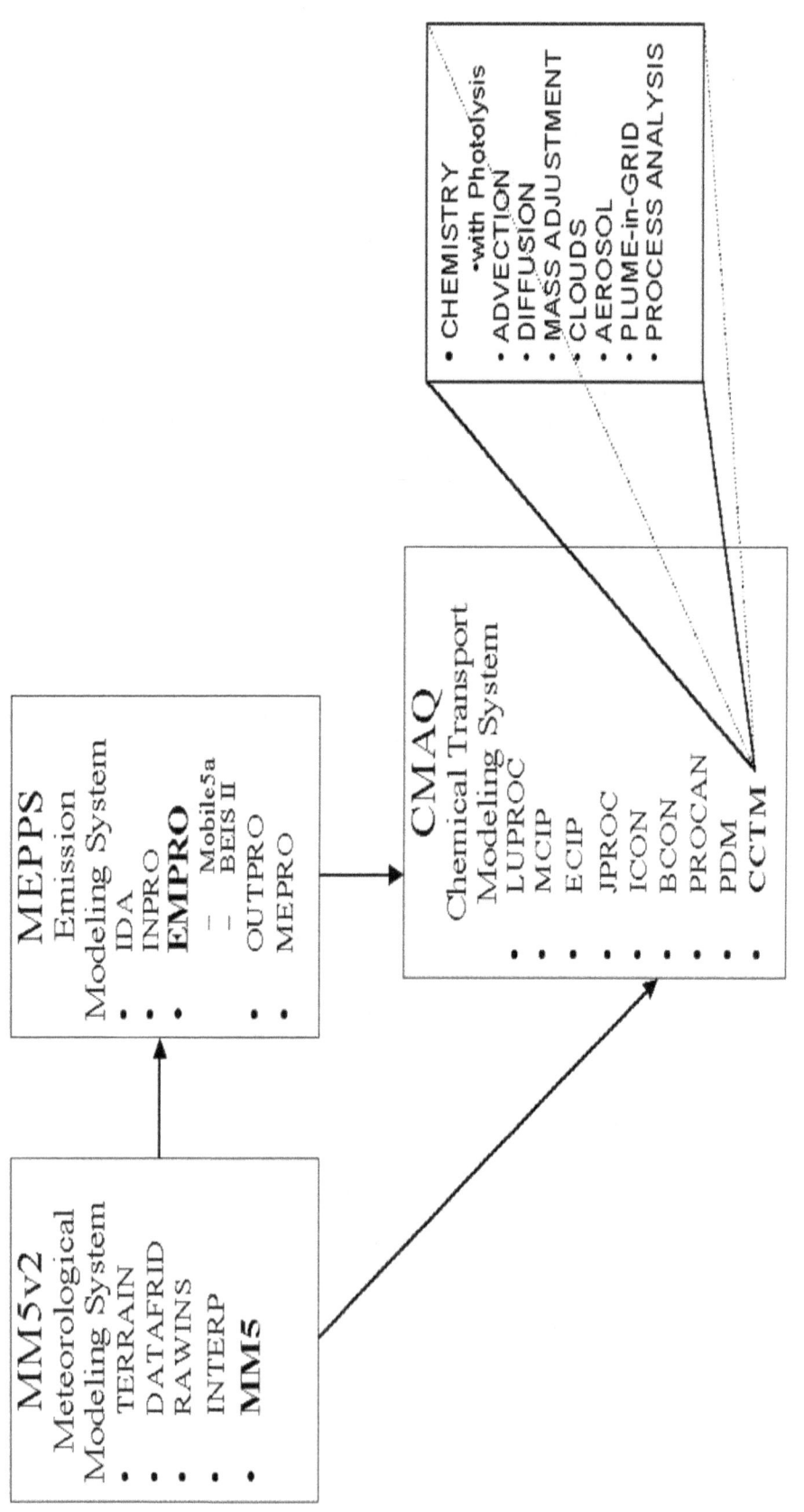

Figure 4.13. Models-3 Relationship Between and Components within the Meteorological, Emission, and Chemistry Transport Environmental Modeling Systems

4.32

Models-3 Framework Components – The Models-3 Framework includes ten major components that are designed to help you use each of these modeling and analysis systems. Each of these components is accessed from the main Models-3 window. A description of the tools that each component provides is as follows:

1. Program Manager – Program Manager allows the user to register, update, and search for executable programs and/or scripts to make them available for use in defining studies within the Study Planner component. During program registration, the user enters characteristics of the program into the framework, including descriptive information on program function, input requirements, output specifications, runtime environment variables, target host computer, and operating system. Once the program or script is registered, this executable can be used in the Study Planner to sequence a series of executions that may depend on previous executions for input data. The user can access and execute programs that are not registered. However, the use of registered programs benefits the user in two ways. First, it enables the user to check and ensure that all mandatory inputs have been specified. Also, it automatically names and registers output files to facilitate tracking output from numerous program executions. Recommended model configurations for standard domains will be preregistered in the system, eliminating the need for the typical user to deal with the details of program registration.

2. Source Code Manager – Use the Source Code Manager to store or retrieve source code for scientific models. It allows you to retrieve a version of a source-code file, change it, and return it to the code archive after the change has been tested. After this file has been returned to the archive, other users can access an updated version of the file. Source Code Manager also tracks historical information on the source code and is used in the compilation process. While the source code should not be changed for most user applications, the CMAQ model and processor source code is included because it is needed for recompilation with different user-specified grid domains. The source code is also needed for model development and testing, which often require source-code modifications.

3. Science Manager – Science Manager allows the user to define globally-shared information on critical model components. In the past, details on horizontal grid coordinates, map projections, vertical layers, and chemical mechanisms have been hardwired and buried within most air-quality-model codes. In Models-3, details on these key science components are entered only once by the user from graphical user interfaces controlled by the Science Manager. The specifications are then saved as named entities in an object-oriented database accessible by all model components. In a typical application, a user would modify an existing set of specifications to define a new modeling domain. More knowledgeable users, however, may use Science Manager to experiment with new model components. To test alternative photochemical mechanisms, for example, the researcher would use Science Manager to edit one of the existing mechanisms, to import a new set of chemical reactions, or to specify new chemical species. Both Regional Acid Deposition Model, Version 2 (RADM-2) and Carbon Bond IV (CB-IV or CB-4) mechanisms are contained within this release of Models-3/CMAQ. If the chemical species for the new mechanism are present in the source-emission profiles, then specifications for this new chemical mechanism would propagate to the emission processing subsystem, and the emission species would be

generated consistent with the new chemical mechanism. Historically, testing a new chemical mechanism in this manner would have involved extensive error-prone software modifications. Science Manager reduces the danger of software errors and reduces the time needed to test alternative science components.

4.   Model Builder – A typical user would access Model Builder to prepare a model for execution in a different location and/or to select an alternative horizontal/vertical grid resolution, and/or a chemical mechanism without the need for reprogramming. A model developer would use Model Builder to interchange science components within a model, to modify details within an existing chemistry mechanism, and/or to experiment with new horizontal and vertical resolutions, coordinate system, nested domain specifications, etc. Model Builder also assists with development of configuration files for creating new model executables from selected existing, modified, and new science process components.

5.   File Converter – The File Converter processes raw input data from ASCII or SAS® files and converts it into formats used in the Models-3 framework (Input/Output Applications Programming Interface [I/O API] and SAS®). The raw data should be delimited by spaces, tabs, or commas. The File Converter can be accessed through the Tools Manager, through Dataset Manager if specific settings are made, or it can be used independently outside of the Models-3 Framework. The most common use for File Converter is to import data, such as monitor data, into Models-3 to analyze or compare with model output using Models-3 visualization packages. File Converter can also be used to import new input data for a model simulation if the standard data files provided with this release are not suitable for your modeling needs. Models-3 also uses the File Converter to convert between Models-3 internal data formats. This is an automatic process that the user does not direct.

6.   Dataset Manager – Dataset Manager provides the user with the capability to register datasets for use with modeling and analysis programs within Models-3. The registration process involves entering the location of the dataset (full path name) and metadata (information about the data, such as spatial-temporal extent and resolution, source of data, time convention, units, etc.) into the Models-3 database. Models-3 follows the Federal Geospatial Metadata Standard for metadata content. The datasets may be located on any network-connected computer system known to the Models-3 system installed at the user's site. Once a dataset is registered, the user can search for the dataset based on its metadata information, file type, etc. Dataset Manager allows the user to view the details of the selected dataset to ensure that the correct one has been selected for use with an application. Dataset registration eliminates the need for the user to type the entire path name each time the dataset is used. Instead, the user can highlight the dataset from a list of candidates that satisfy the search criteria specified by the user. Models-3 will automatically move selected data to the host where it is needed for a model execution. Dataset Manager also provides standard capabilities, such as deleting, copying, archiving, and restoring files and metadata.

7.   Strategy Manager – With Strategy Manager, the user can estimate future-year point-, area-, and mobile-source emissions and determine the relative effectiveness of specified control scenarios. The user may adjust pollutant growth factors and emissions-control factors to perform "what if" analyses for EPA regions, states, counties, or user-defined study areas. By applying estimated yearly emission growth factors from the Emissions Growth and Assessment System, control efficiency, rule effectiveness, and rule penetration factors to

the EPA 1990 base-year emissions inventory, the Strategy Manager estimates future year (1991 to 2010) emissions for carbon monoxide, nitrogen oxide, particulate matter up to 10 microns, sulfur dioxide, and volatile organic compounds. Strategy Manager is based on EPA's Multiple Projection System. An input data processor will be added to process the Emission Inventory Improvement Program (URL http://www.epa.gov/oar/oaqps/eiip) data format after it is finalized.

8. Tools Manager – Tools Manager provides access to a variety of visualization, statistical analysis, and emissions processing tools that are registered with the Models-3 framework. The tools that are accessible are Vis5D, Text Editor, MEPPS, PAVE, Statistical Analysis System (SAS)®, ARCInfo®, IDA, and VisDriver. MEPPS is an advanced tool that can be used for specifying emissions preparation and processing emissions details. MEPPS can be used to import emissions-inventory data, perform QC on emissions-inventory data, and reformat or subset data for the user-specified modeling domain. Mobile emissions are calculated using Mobile 5a emission factors, and biogenic emissions are calculated using the Biogenic Emissions Inventory System (BEIS2). The system used in MEPPS for the main emissions processing requires the user to have Arc/Info® and SAS® licenses for operation, which are not included with Models-3.

9. Study Planner – Study Planner allows the user to define a study and control the execution of its associated models and processors. A study is a collection of plans and properties necessary to describe and perform one or more environmental modeling analyses. A plan is a collection of information defining dataset and program interdependencies and the sequence of execution. Study Planner gathers much of its information from the Program Manager and Dataset Manager registration data. The relationship between a program (node) and its required and optional datasets (links) is user-defined through the process of constructing and annotating a graphical diagram with simple drag-and-click mouse operations. Once a plan is constructed and its graphical diagram fully annotated with desired input datasets and options, the plan can be executed. User-specified program options are entered by editing program-environment variables. Studies and associated plans are named entities that are saved in the system database. Therefore, a typical user can start with an existing study plan provided by the model developer and simply change the dataset annotations by selecting, through a file browser, appropriate datasets needed for execution. The Study Planner provides capabilities to create new studies, copy and modify existing studies, and delete existing studies.

10. Framework Administrator – This component allows the Models-3 framework administrator to register, update, and delete users, hosts, devices, compilers, and operating systems as well as establish access roles and dataset types and perform other administrative tasks.

Models-3 Major System Functions – The Models-3 framework helps you build and execute air-quality simulation models and visualize their results. The following are some examples of tasks that you could perform with Models-3:

•   Prepare required emission and meteorological inputs for air-quality modeling studies

- Prepare emission control strategies by defining new input data sets or by modifying existing emissions data to represent the strategies of interest

- Prepare source emission estimates for future-year scenarios based on projected economic sector and population growth

- Execute 3D dynamic meteorological models to provide detailed consistent meteorological fields required to drive air-quality-model simulations

- Define your own computational domain for air-quality-model simulations

- Select or define alternative chemistry mechanisms and vertical and horizontal grid resolutions for your simulations without rewriting or modifying the source code

- Manage and organize large collections of model executions and associated data.

Models-3 also helps in model-development tasks of assembling, testing, and evaluating science-process components and their impact on CMAQ chemistry-transport model (CCTM) predictions. Models-3 can do this by facilitating the interchange of process modules and the execution of the modeling system. In addition to the capability needed for the application users, the Models-3 system provides critical functionality for model development by making it possible to:

- Modify the horizontal or vertical resolution, coordinate system, or map projection of the CCTM without rewriting source code and Interface with different meteorological models to drive the CCTM

- Insert a new chemical mechanism or modify an existing one in the CCTM without rewriting the code

- Test new science formulations and numerical solvers via interchange of modular components in the CCTM

- Quantify the contribution of various physical and chemical processes to the simulated pollutant concentrations using process analysis

- Quantify the effect of a specific model component on the CCTM predictions by allowing the substitution of a no-operation module for individual science components

- Perform model-sensitivity analysis, evaluation, and application studies on a variety of computing platforms.

4.3.2.3 Selected Applications of Models-3

A project is underway to apply the Models-3 framework, with the MM5 meteorological model and the CMAQ photochemistry/transport model, to an area of Southern Ontario, Canada, centered on the City of Hamilton (Boulton et al. 1999). Considerable effort is being devoted to adaptation of the most recent Canadian emission inventory data (the 1995 CAC Inventory) for use within Models-3. Concurrent with this work is a Canadian research project to improve the chemistry and aerosol modules of CMAQ, which will enhance CMAQ's capability to simulate fine particulate matter. Preliminary simulations have already been performed and future simulations are planned once the emission-inventory work and the modification of the chemistry and aerosol modules are complete. In addition, detailed monitoring of air pollutants has been undertaken for a high ozone and particulate matter episode in the summer of 1999. The resultant temporalized and speciated monitoring data will be used in model-validation efforts.

4.3.3 Multimedia Integration Modeling System

4.3.3.1 Purpose and General Attributes of MIMS

The EPA's ORD is embarking on a long term project to develop a MIMS. The system is being designed to represent the transport and fate of nutrients and chemical stressors in the environment over multiple scales. MIMS is intended to improve the environmental-management community's ability to evaluate the impact of air-quality and watershed-management practices on stream and estuarine conditions. The system will provide a computer-based problem-solving environment for testing our understanding of multimedia (atmosphere, land, water) environmental problems, such as the movement of chemicals through the hydrologic cycle, or the response of aquatic ecological systems to land-use change, with initial emphasis on the fish-health endpoint. The design will attempt to combine the state-of-the-art in computer science, system design, and numerical analysis (i.e., object-oriented analysis and design, parallel processing, advanced numerical libraries) with the latest advancements in process level science (process chemistry, hydrology, atmospheric, and ecological science). The problem-solving environment will embrace the watershed/airshed approach to environmental management and build upon the latest technologies for environmental monitoring and geographic representation. The MIMS team will promote a common and open modeling framework for the university and government modeling communities and will be open to cooperative arrangements with private partners, where appropriate.

4.3.3.2 Descriptive Summary of MIMS

The challenges of today's environmental problems far exceed what any one group or agency can expect to resolve; thus, MIMS will adopt an open framework (non-proprietary) technology approach to facilitate the combination of individual science components into collaborating multi-disciplinary, multi-scale modeling and assessment tools. The goal is to develop the technology foundation and guidelines to enable MIMS components to operate in a cross-platform computing environment (from Personal Computers to networks of workstations to scalable parallel computers) with transparent distributed data access. Therefore, an object-oriented analysis/design approach has been selected, MIMS development, which will fully meet Models 2000 goals related to model testing, evaluation, and documentation. In order to handle inconsistent time and space scales for intermedia information exchanges and to more closely integrate geospatial analysis and science process models, research will be conducted on 1) more powerful data models that embed information about the grid and coordinate systems as part of the data object, and 2) intelligent agents for data exchange among media.

MIMS will provide a solid foundation for agency activities in the OW, such as the evaluation of ecological assimilative capabilities in the calculation of TMDLs, or in the design of protection zones around public water supplies. The air-quality and deposition components directly support the OAQPS state implementation planning process for attainment of the National Ambient Air Quality Standards (NAAQS). And through linkage of air and water components, MIMS will enable the assessment of the cost/benefits associated with Clean Air Act requirements for nitrogen control as they relate to nitrogen loading in the watershed.

The MIMS project has been initiated to develop a problem-solving software framework to support ecosystem modeling and environmental health assessment. The long-term objectives of developing MIMS are to:

- Foster and establish a "community approach" to a multistressor, multimedia, multiscale environmental modeling system

- Foster active participation in the community development of scientific, technical, computational, and procedural guidance

- Construct and maintain an open-architecture software system that enables (1) data access and management, (2) development, linkage, and execution of simulation modules at various spatial and temporal scales, and (3) visualization, analysis, and interpretation of model outputs

- Incorporate and further the development of state-of-the-science process and component modules

- Develop innovative techniques to resolve spatial and temporal mismatches and multiple-scale flexibility

- Develop efficient computational approaches to meet increased demands of complex, multiscale, multimedia, multi-dimensional environmental models

- Develop dynamic, intelligent computer interfaces to assist users in accessing and synthesizing data, information, and knowledge related to environmental-assessment issues

- Incorporate links to effects and activity-pattern databases and socioeconomic, demographic, and climatic predictive forcing functions to assemble problem-solving methodologies.

Figure 4.14 presents the MIMS conceptual structure, represented as a description of entities and a diagram (which uses an informal notation) among these entities. The lines on the diagram can be read as sentences starting with the entity at the origin of the line, followed by the text along the line, and finally the text at the destination of the line. For example, the line between the Session Manager and the System Administration Manager at the left side of the diagram could be read as "Session Manager invokes System Administration Manager."

Five major science components have been identified for MIMS, as illustrated in Figure 4.15: atmosphere, Basin Land, Basin Surface Water, Macrobiota, and Subsurface. The central scientific focus will be on a physically-based representation of the convective/advective transport of solutes and particles at multiple scales and media (air-land-water), within a framework supporting fate and transformation processes, and ecosystem response modeling. Primary transport and transformation will include accurate representation of the hydrologic cycle, biogeochemical cycles, and the resultant advective flow, accounting for the water budget, and mass conservation of the chemical and nutrient budgets. Elements of the hydrologic cycle of particular importance for ecosystem assessments are precipitation, interception, evapotranspiration, overland and channel flow, subsurface unsaturated and saturated flow, soil, aquifer, and snowpack storage, and the dynamics between groundwater and surface-water hydrology in streamflow generation. Accurate representation of the nitrogen and phosphorous cycles in both the gaseous and sedimentary forms, including natural fluxes and man-made sources and sinks (chemical transformations, deposition, biotic uptake/release) of nutrients and chemical stressors, is also being addressed. Soil, sedimentary, and gaseous forms of organics and key metals of interest will be incorporated over the long term.

4.3.3.3 Selected Applications of MIMS

In the shorter-term, a comprehensive ecosystem exposure-assessment case study will be constructed to measure aquatic ecosystem health, with fish health and water quality as the initial endpoints. Coupling multiple environmental models will introduce many challenges, such as atmospheric-terrestrial interactions, spatial and temporal-scale discrepancies, non-continuous grid structuring, and database handling.

A Research Implementation Plan is under development for planned peer review. A broad conceptual model of the cross-media watershed dynamics is being prepared in collaboration with the academic community. A conceptual model was developed during FY 1999 to serve as the design basis for planning process-oriented monitoring and model development. The next 3 years will target the development of a proof-of-concept prototype by the end of FY 2002, implementing the atmospheric-hydrospheric foundation and selected ecological functionality for multimedia modeling in the Albemarle-Pamilico basin, including the Neuse River, and associated airshed of influence. Once the open framework object-oriented approach has been proven, the effort will continue toward a prototype beta version by the end of FY 2005, including the nutrients nitrogen and phosphorus, sediments endpoints. The fish health ecological endpoint is planned for progressively more detailed implementation through FY 2005, along with management and economic. After 2 years of beta testing and verification against available field data, the MIMS will be scheduled for public release at the end of FY 2008.

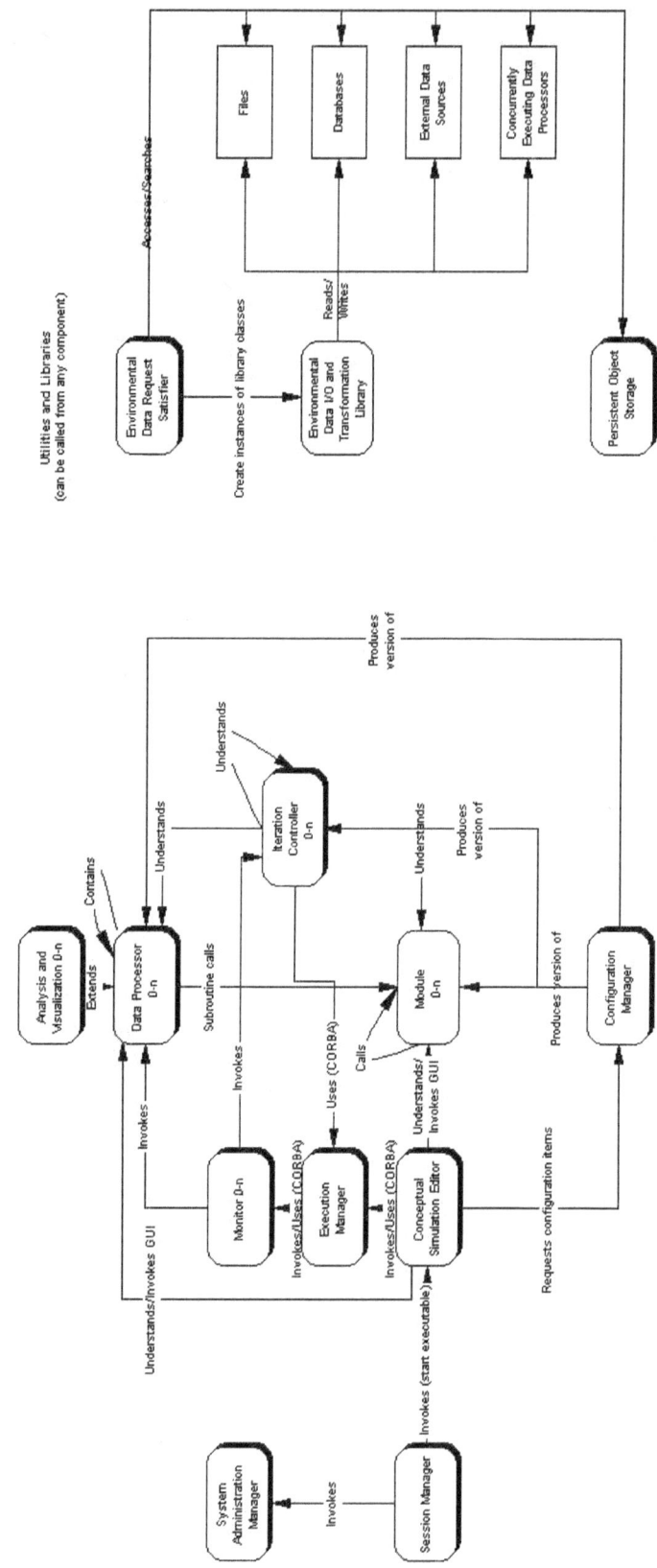

Notes: "0-n" indicates that an arbitrary number of entities would be present.
Shadows denote entities that contain one or more computational applications.
Text in parentheses along the links indicates the communication mechanism used.

Figure 4.14 MIMS Conceptual Structure, Represented as a Description of Entities and a Diagram Among These Entities

4.40

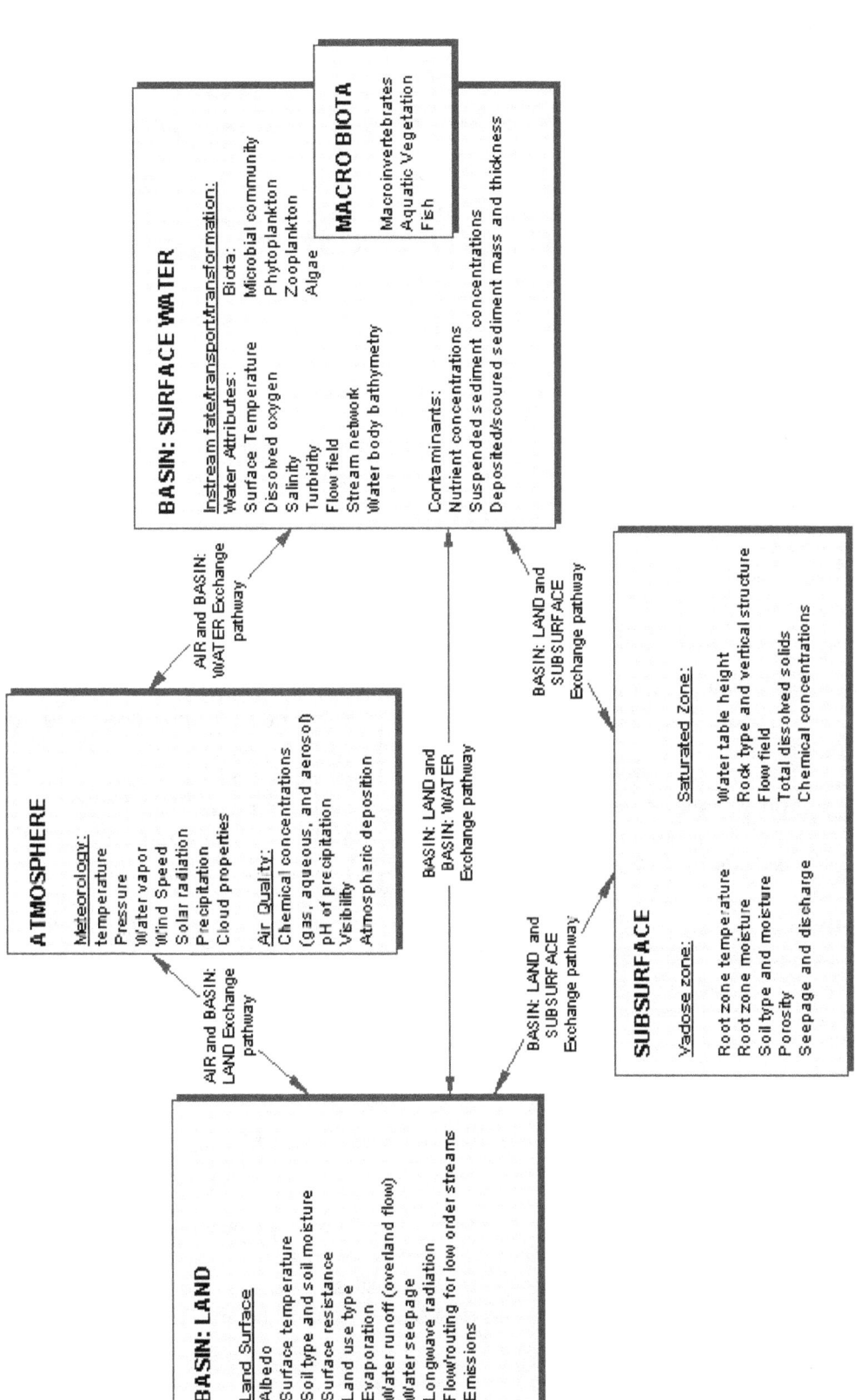

Figure 4.15. Five Major Science Components of MIMS: Atmosphere, Basin Land, Basin Surface Water, Macrobiota, and Subsurface

4.41

4.3.4 Total Risk Information Model

4.3.4.1 Purpose and General Attributes of TRIM

TRIM is intended to provide EPA-OAQPS with a modeling system for assessing human health and ecological risks resulting from multimedia, multipathway exposure to air pollutants. It is designed to be scientifically defensible (e.g., conservation of pollutant mass), flexible (modular in design, flexible in temporal and spatial scale), and usable by OAQPS and stakeholders (easily accessible, clear, and transparent). Toward this end, TRIM currently satisfies several of the desired attributes stated as goals of any framework:

- Platform-independence
- Version 1 implemented in Java (uses some Fortran/C libraries)
- Has been executed on Unix, Solaris, and Win95/98/NT
- Feedback: Within TRIM.FaTE, feedback between compartments is incorporated
- Monitoring data: Methodology allows for use of monitoring data at any step
- Explicitly address parameter uncertainty and variability
- QA/QC Capabilities
- Plug-and-play: User can make use of libraries of algorithms, property types, compartments.

4.3.4.2 Descriptive Summary of TRIM

EPA's OAQPS has the responsibility for the hazardous and criteria air pollutant [a] programs described by Sections 112 and 108 of CAA. OAQPS recognized the need for improved fate and transport, exposure, and risk modeling tools in response to aspects of these programs that require an evaluation of health risks and environmental effects associated with air pollutant exposures, as well as scientific recommendations of the National Academy of Sciences (NRC 1994), the Presidential/Congressional Commission on Risk Assessment and Risk Management (CRARM 1997), and Agency guidelines and policies. To support evaluations with a scientifically sound, flexible, and user-friendly methodology, the TRIM, a time series modeling system with multimedia capabilities for assessing human health and ecological risks from hazardous and criteria air pollutants, is being developed. The TRIM design includes three modules: the Environmental Fate, Transport, and Ecological Exposure module, TRIM.FaTE; the human Exposure-Event module, TRIM.Expo; and, the Risk Characterization module, TRIM.Risk.

The first TRIM module to be developed, TRIM.FaTE, is a spatial compartmental mass balance model that describes the movement and transformation of pollutants over time through a user-

---

(a) Hazardous air pollutants (HAPs) are those pollutants listed under CAA section 112(b); currently, there are 188 HAPs. Criteria air pollutants are air pollutants for which national ambient air quality standards have been established under the CAA; at present, they are particulate matter, ozone, carbon monoxide, nitrogen oxides, sulfur dioxide, and lead.

defined, bounded system that includes both biotic and abiotic compartments. TRIM.FaTE, the emphasis for which is air pollutants for which non-inhalation exposures are important, generates both media concentrations relevant to human pollutant exposures and exposure estimates relevant to ecological risk assessment. The Exposure-Event module, TRIM.Expo, can receive input from TRIM.FaTE or from air-quality models or monitoring data. In TRIM.Expo, human exposures are evaluated by tracking population groups referred to as "cohorts" and their inhalation and ingestion through time and space. An overarching feature of the TRIM design is the analysis of uncertainty and variability. A two-stage approach for providing this feature to the user has been developed: (1) sensitivity analyses, (2) Monte Carlo methods (e.g., for refined assessment of the impact of the critical parameters).

The TRIM is being developed using an object-oriented approach. There has been much discussion in the software engineering literature, such as Booch (1993), on the benefits of this approach, including increased software extensibility, reusability, and maintainability. The essence of object-oriented software development is that concepts, such as a volume element, are represented as a unit that contains internal data (e.g., the boundaries of a volume element) and operations on the data (e.g., computation of volume), and that one class of objects (e.g., volume element with vertical sides) can be a specialization of another class of objects (e.g., volume element). Being able to specialize classes of objects allows general functionality to be shared by several specialized classes. The TRIM's representation of the outdoor environment (with volume elements that contain compartments) and the development of associated graphical user interfaces are well suited for an object-oriented treatment.

The TRIM computer framework and TRIM.FaTE module have been developed primarily, but not entirely, in the Java programming language. Some parts of TRIM.FaTE, such as the differential equation solver, and other TRIM modules, such as TRIM.Expo, ultimately will be implemented in the FORTRAN or other programming languages. As shown in Figure 4.16, the TRIM computer system architecture is complex but flexible, allowing it to be applied in developing each of the different TRIM modules. The architecture components used to describe TRIM are classified as those that primarily provide (1) functionality (rectangles), and (2) data (ovals). However, each of the components, except for external data sources, provide both functionality and data. This figure is designed to represent the relationships within the TRIM computer framework rather than the data flow within the system.

The TRIM Core component primarily provides services required by multiple architectural components or integrates those components. Projects in TRIM are used to store all information pertinent to an individual assessment. A project contains "scenarios," where each scenario contains a description of the outdoor environment being simulated, populations being studied, and model parameters, such as the simulation time step. Each project also displays the information it contains and allows the user to change that information. In some cases, the information display and manipulation functions of a project rely on a TRIM Core functionality, such as the property editor. Each TRIM module, such as TRIM.FaTE, is a component that allows for simulation or analysis. Where required, modules also provide specialized graphical user interfaces that support their functionality.

4.43

A substantial amount of relatively static information is required to assess multimedia chemical fate and transport and subsequent exposures and effects on selected populations. For instance, static information includes the measured properties of chemicals that change infrequently or the boundaries of a study region that might stay constant for years. Because of the static nature of this information and because a large amount of static information may be needed for a single assessment, users can store such information in TRIM libraries. Users can then easily reuse

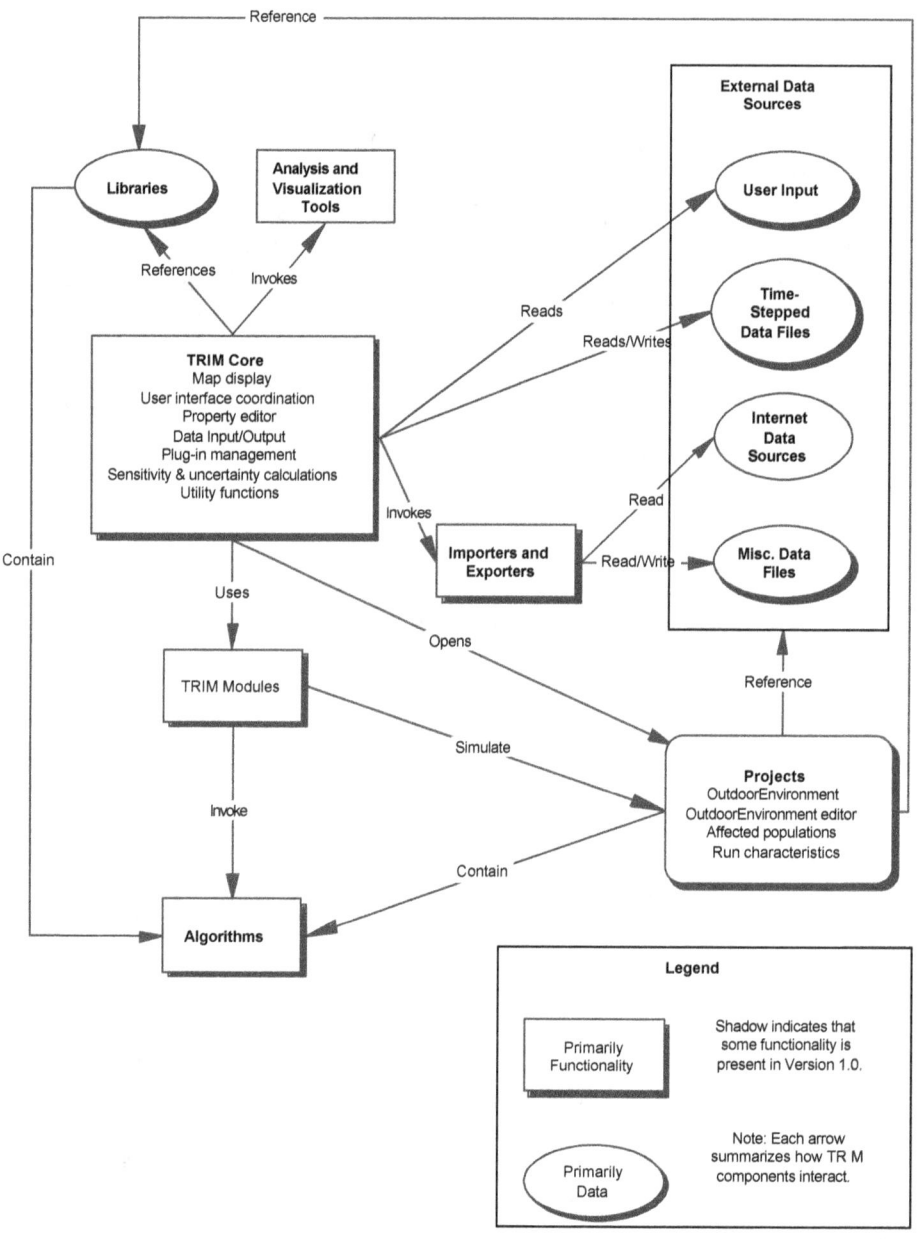

Figure 4.16. TRIM Computer System Architecture

selected information from a library in future projects. Changes may be made to the library over time to ensure that the most current science is used in assessments. However, when a user creates a project that accesses information from a library, a copy of the information is made to protect the project from future changes to the library.

The TRIM.FaTE module uses a number of chemical fate and transport algorithms that compute chemical-transfer coefficients between and chemical-transformation coefficients within compartments. As new chemicals, ecosystems, and relationships are studied, new algorithms will be required. In anticipation of this need, TRIM.FaTE has been designed to allow users to add algorithms. The algorithms are stored in libraries and can be applied to various projects, as designated by the user. Specifically, a user can manually assign algorithms stored in libraries to links or can request that TRIM.FaTE assign applicable algorithms based on the compartments that are connected by a link. For instance, some algorithms might only be applicable for transfer from surface water to fish. Even when TRIM.FaTE assigns algorithms, the user can review the assignments and make changes before the simulation starts. Before or after a simulation, the user can export the simulation scenario and its results (if available) to a set of hypertext markup language (HTML) files. These HTML files show which algorithms were used for each link and the formulation of each algorithm.

Given the diversity of potential applications of TRIM, data required to address those applications, and formats used for storing that data, it is difficult to construct a computer framework that provides all potentially required capabilities. The TRIM architecture addresses this issue in several ways. The architecture allows the user to add data importers and exporters in a relatively easy manner, as needed. Data importers read non-TRIM data sets and create and/or set appropriate TRIM objects and properties. For instance, Version 1.0 contains a data importer that can read a text file describing volume elements and can create the corresponding elements in a TRIM project. Another data importer can read a textual description of algorithms, compartments, chemicals, and sources and can create the corresponding objects in a TRIM library. Data exporters can write TRIM configurations and results in a format that is suitable for use by another computer program or for interactive review. Version 1.0 can export the configuration of a simulation scenario and its results to HTML files and simulation results to a text file that can be imported by Microsoft® Excel. Future data importers and exporters could provide many other capabilities. Examples include reading data produced by a GIS (e.g., SHAPE files) and interpolating values to TRIM volume elements, writing results in a format that could be further processed by a GIS, importing information directly from a web site or database, and transferring results to a statistical package that is executing concurrently with TRIM. To provide additional flexibility, future versions of TRIM may allow knowledgeable users to apply data importers and exporters that users develop without modifying TRIM.

The TRIM.FaTE module, in specific, allows users to provide environmental data in binary files that can be read as needed by a TRIM.FaTE simulation. This streamlines the use of large data sets, such as hourly temperatures or concentrations over a 30-year period. Binary files can also be used for storing TRIM.FaTE results. The TRIM Core supports reading data from and writing data to file formats that are based on the Environmental Decision Support System/Models-3 I/O API (Coats 1998). The I/O API format can be easily read and written from several programming languages, is platform-independent, is suitable for large data sets, is self-describing (i.e., contains information about variables and time periods contained in the file), and is computationally efficient. Instead, simulation results can be easily exported to Microsoft® Excel or other analysis packages. In the future, TRIM will include some analysis and visualization capabilities and may allow users to develop and plug in additional capabilities.

4.3.4.3 Selected Applications of TRIM

As mentioned earlier, TRIM is intended to support assessment activities for both the criteria and hazardous air pollutant programs of OAQPS. As a result of the greater level of effort expended by the Agency on assessment activities for criteria air pollutants, these activities are generally more widely known. To improve the public understanding of the hazardous air pollutant (or air toxics) program, the Agency published an overview of the air toxics program in July 1999 (64 FR 38705–38740). Air-toxics assessment activities (National Air Toxics Assessment [NATA]) are described as one of the program's key components.[a] The NATA includes both national- and local-scale activities. The TRIM system is intended to provide tools in support of local-scale assessment activities, including multimedia analyses.

One of the Agency's most immediate needs for TRIM comes in the Residual Risk Program in which there are statutory deadlines within the next 2 to 9 years for risk-based emissions-standards decisions. As described in the *Residual Risk Report to Congress* (EPA 1999a), TRIM is intended to improve upon the Agency's ability to perform multipathway human-health risk assessments and ecological risk assessments for HAPs with the potential for multimedia environmental distribution. Another important upcoming use for TRIM is in exposure assessment in support of the review of the ozone NAAQS. The TRIM.Expo and

> **EXAMPLES OF TRIM APPLICATIONS**
>
> A human health or ecological assessment of multimedia, multipathway risks associated with mercury emissions from one or several local sources could be performed using all three modules in the TRIM system.
>
> An assessment of human-health risks associated with air emissions of a criteria air pollutant (e.g., ozone) or one or several volatile HAPs in a metropolitan area could be developed using an external air model or ambient concentration data from fixed-site monitors coupled with TRIM.Expo and TRIM.Risk.

(a) Within the air toxics program, these activities are intended to help EPA identify areas of concern (e.g., pollutants, locations, or sources), characterize risks, and track progress toward meeting the Agency's overall air toxics program goals, as well as the risk-based goals of the various activities and initiatives within the program, such as residual risk assessments and the Integrated Urban Air Toxics Strategy. More specifically, NATA activities include expansion of air toxics monitoring, improvements and periodic updates to emissions inventories, national- and local-scale air-quality modeling, multimedia and exposure modeling (including modeling that considers stationary and mobile sources), continued research on health effects of and exposures to both ambient and indoor air, and use and improvement of exposure and assessment tools. These activities are intended to provide the Agency with improved characterizations of air toxics risk and of risk reductions resulting from emissions-control standards and initiatives for both stationary and mobile source programs.

TRIM.Risk modules augmented with external air-quality monitoring data and models are intended to support this type of criteria pollutant assessment as well as risk assessments for non-multimedia HAPs.

Consistent with the phased plan of TRIM development, the application of TRIM will also be initiated in a phased approach. With the further development of the TRIM modules in 2000 and 2001, EPA will begin to use the modules to contribute to or support CAA exposure and risk assessments. These initial applications also will contribute to model evaluation. The earliest TRIM activities are expected to include the use of TRIM.FaTE side-by-side (at a comparable level of detail) with the existing multimedia methodology[a] in risk assessments of certain multimedia HAPs (e.g., mercury) under the Residual Risk Program. As TRIM.Expo is developed to accommodate inhalation modeling of HAPs and after it has undergone testing, OAQPS plans to initially run it side-by-side (at a comparable level of detail) with EPA's existing inhalation exposure model, HEM (Human Exposure Model [EPA 1986]). When TRIM.Risk has been completed, it will be used, as appropriate, in risk assessments for both criteria and hazardous air pollutants.

In later years, OAQPS intends to use TRIM and the TRIM modules in a variety of activities including (1) residual risk assessments using TRIM.FaTE, TRIM.Expo, and TRIM.Risk, in combinations appropriate to the environmental distribution characteristics of the HAPs being assessed, (2) urban scale assessments on case-study cities as part of the Integrated Urban Air Toxics Strategy, and (3) exposure and risk assessments of criteria air pollutants (e.g., ozone, carbon monoxide) in support of NAAQS reviews.

4.3.5 GENII-2

4.3.5.1 Purpose and General Attributes of GENII-2

The GENII computer code was developed at PNNL to incorporate the internal dosimetry models recommended by ICRP and the radiological risk estimating procedures of Federal Guidance Report 13 into updated versions of existing models for analyzing environmental pathways. The resulting environmental-dosimetry computer codes are compiled in the GENII Environmental Dosimetry System. The GENII system was developed to provide a state-of-the-art, technically peer-reviewed, documented set of programs for calculating radiation dose and risk from radionuclides released to the environment. The codes were designed with the flexibility to accommodate input parameters for a wide variety of generic sites. GENII Version 1 was released in 1988. A new version of the codes, GENII Version 2, has been developed for the U.S. Environmental Protection Administration, incorporating improved transport models, exposure options, dose and risk estimation, and user

---

(a) In support of the *Mercury Report to Congress* (EPA 1997) and the *Study of Hazardous Air Pollutant Emissions from Electric Utility Steam Generating Units -- Final Report to Congress* (EPA 1998), the Agency relied upon the Indirect Exposure Methodology, which has recently been updated and is now termed the Multiple Pathways of Exposure methodology (EPA 1999b). This methodology is being used in initial assessment activities for the Residual Risk Program (EPA 1999a).

interfaces. The new version is specifically designed to function within FRAMES, a framework that allows GENII to execute with, and provide inputs to, other related programs.

The GENII system includes the capabilities for calculating radiation doses following chronic and acute releases. Radionuclide transport via air, water, or biological activity may be considered. Air-transport options include both puff and plume models, and each allow use of an effective stack height or calculation of plume rise from buoyant or momentum effects (or both). Building wake effects can be included in acute atmospheric release scenarios. The code provides radiation dose and/or risk estimates for health effects to individuals or populations; radiation dose may be reported as either effective dose equivalent or organ dose, and health risk may be reported as cancer incidence or fatalities. GENII Version 2 uses cancer-risk factors from Federal Guidance Report 13 to estimate risk to specific organs or tissues.

Data entry is accomplished via interactive, window-driven user interfaces. Default exposure and consumption parameters are provided for both the average (population) and maximum individual; however, these may be modified by the user. Source-term information may be entered as radionuclide release quantities for transport scenarios or as initial radionuclide concentrations in environmental media (air, water, soil). For input of released or initial concentrations, decay of parent radionuclides and ingrowth of radioactive decay products may be considered before the start of and during the exposure scenario. A single code run can accommodate unlimited numbers of radionuclides, including the source term, and any radionuclides that accumulate from decay of the parent because the system works sequentially on individual decay chains.

The code package also provides interfaces, through FRAMES, for external calculations of atmospheric dispersion, geohydrology, biotic transport, and surface-water transport. Target populations are identified by direction and distance (radial or cartesian grids for Version 2) for individuals, populations, and for intruders into contained sources.

A stochastic edition of GENII Version 1, named GENII-S, was developed for the Waste Isolation Pilot Plant assessments by Sandia National Laboratory (Leigh et al. 1992). GENII Version 2 is completely stochastic, using the FRAMES Sensitivity/Uncertainty Multimedia Modeling Module (SUM³) driver.

4.3.5.2 Descriptive Summary of GENII-2

GENII is intended to be used as a general-purpose package for estimating the consequences of radionuclides released into the environment. Available release scenarios include chronic and acute releases to water or to air (ground level or elevated sources), and initial contamination of soil or surfaces. GENII implements models developed for NRC for surface-water transport. GENII does not explicitly include modules for performing groundwater transport calculations; however the FRAMES system, in which GENII functions, allows addition of other computer modules to the GENII system. Exposure pathways include direct exposure via water (swimming, boating, and fishing), soil (surface and buried sources), air (semi-infinite cloud and finite-cloud geometries), inhalation, and ingestion pathways. Special models are included for tritium and carbon-14; the tritium model includes exposure via skin absorption. An additional capability for releases of radon isotopes is planned.

GENII Version 1 implemented dosimetry models recommended by the ICRP in Publications 26, 30, and 48 and approved for use by DOE Order 5400.5. GENII Version 2 implements these models plus those of ICRP Publications 56 through 72 and the related risk factors published in Federal Guidance Report 13. Risk factors in the form of EPA developed "slope factors" are also included. At the discretion of the user, different dose and risk approaches may be compared and contrasted. These dosimetry and risk models are considered to be "state of the art" by the international radiation-protection community and have been adopted by most national and international organizations as their standard dosimetry methodology.

The GENII Version 2 system consists of four independent atmospheric models, one surface-water model, three independent environmental accumulation models, one exposure module, and one dose/risk module, each with a specific user-interface code. The computer programs are of several types: user interfaces (interactive, window-driven programs to assist the user with scenario generation and data input), internal and external dose-factor libraries, the environmental-dosimetry programs, and FRAMES-supplied file-viewing routines. For maximum flexibility, the code has been divided into several interrelated, but separate, exposure and dose calculations. The components of the system communicate with each other through a series of intermediate data files. Each of the intermediate files is accessible to the user through the FRAMES data-visualization utilities. Each module is also connected to the sensitivity/uncertainty driver SUM^3, which allows assignment of distributions to all input parameters and which will run the entire system in a Monte Carlo fashion.

The source input module is provided by FRAMES. The four atmospheric dispersion models are available for use, depending on the nature of the problem to be solved and the quality of available data. The acute and chronic gaussian-plume models can be run on either hourly or compiled joint--frequency data on wind speed, direction, and stability. The acute and chronic lagrangian-puff models require more-detailed hourly inputs, but provide more detailed transport-modeling options. Dry and wet deposition, for gases and various types of particles, is estimated in each case. Utility programs are included to translate several types of available meteorological data into GENII input files. The water-transport model for single surfaces incorporates simple and complex submodels for rivers, lakes, and coastal regions and may be used for simulating either accidents or routine releases. As noted, GENII does not include a groundwater transport module, but others that function within FRAMES may be used if desired. The three terrestrial transport models are tailored for chronic accumulation, accidental releases, and defined initial contaminant distributions in surface or deep soils. The human intake module allows customization of the exposure of individuals to environmental contamination, up to 15 categories of pathways (with as many as 4 pathways per category) for up to 6 age groups. The dose and risk module includes the older ICRP models (for comparison with DOE and NRC regulations), the newer ICRP models, and risk estimation using EPA slope factors, dose-to-risk conversion factors, or the latest Federal Guidance Report 13 methods. The various impacts modules are provided by FRAMES to manipulate, summarize, and organize output as desired.

Both GENII versions were developed under QA plans based on the American National Standards Institute (ANSI) standard NQA-1 as implemented in the PNNL Quality Assurance Manual. All steps of the code development have been documented and tested, and hand calculations have verified the code's implementation of major transport and exposure pathways for a subset of the radionuclide library. A collection of hand calculations and other verification activities is available. A comprehensive test plan has been developed, and testing is underway.

GENII Version 1 has been included in the International Atomic Energy Agency's VAMP project (VAlidation of Model Predictions - an acronym for the Coordinated Research Program on Validation of Models for the Transfer of Radionuclides in Terrestrial, Urban, and Aquatic Environments), an international effort to compare environmental radionuclide transport models with measured environmental data. Results for test scenario CB (based on environmental measurements following the Chernobyl accident) indicated that dose estimates from GENII were comparable to, although slightly higher than, those of other participating models, which is consistent with its primary function as a prospective analysis tool. The models included in the code have been validated to various degrees by additional studies; however, these have not been compared directly to output from the code.

GENII Version 2 requires Windows 95 or 98 and Pentium processors and disk storage in excess of 20 Mbytes. The overall system design is documented in the GENII Version 2 Software Design Document.[a] Specific instruction on the use of FRAMES and the SUM^3 processor is available in electronic and print forms.[b] A Users' Guide explains user interactions with the GENII modules themselves.[c] A series of example cases is available electronically; these are described in Napier.[d] Electronic documentation of GENII Version 2 is available, and the code, documentation, and users' manuals will be made available through the Internet by EPA in the near future. Codes and documentation are also available on compact disk.

(a) Napier, B.A., D.L. Strenge, J.V. Ramsdell, Jr., P.W. Eslinger, and C.F. Fosmire. 1999. *GENII Version 2 Software Design Document*, Pacific Northwest National Laboratory, Richland Washington (Draft).

(b)Gelston, G. M., M. A. Pelton, K. J. Castleton, B. L. Hoopes, R. Y Taira, P. W. Eslinger, G. Whelan, P. D. Meyer, and B. A. Napier. 1998. *GENII Version 2 Sensitivity/Uncertainty Multimedia Modeling Module Users' Guidance*, Pacific Northwest National Laboratory, Richland Washington. (Draft).

(c) Napier, B.A. 1999. *GENII Version 2 Users' Guide*. Pacific Northwest National Laboratory, Richland, Washington (Draft).

(d) Napier, B.A. 1999. *GENII Version 2 Example Calculation Descriptions*. Pacific Northwest National Laboratory, Richland, Washington (Draft).

4.3.5.3 Selected Applications of GENII-2

Since GENII Version 2 is a new system still under development, there is no history of applications yet. Because GENII Version 2 is based on FRAMES and is an extension of the FRAMES capabilities, many of the FRAMES applications are similar to those envisioned for GENII Version 2. However, GENII Version 1.485 (the version currently distributed by the Radiation Safety Information Computational Center, the International Atomic Energy Agency, and PNNL) has been used in numerous applications around the world, and it is reasonable to assume that future applications could be similar.

- **Environmental Compliance** – The GENII 1.485 system is used at DOE's Hanford Site to show compliance with environmental regulations. The code is the primary approved code of the Hanford Environmental Dose Overview Program at Hanford (Schreckhise et al. 1993), and is used for all public dose calculations related to the Hanford Site annual environmental monitoring reports (e.g., Poston et al. 2000). GENII Version 2 is under consideration by EPA for NESHAPS-related calculations.

- **Environmental Impact Statements** – The GENII 1.485 system has been used for evaluating alternatives in a number of environmental analyses, such as those for the decommissioning of surplus production reactors (DOE 1989), or the production of medical radioisotopes (DOE 1996).

- **Regulatory Analyses** – The GENII 1.485 system has been used to evaluate a number of generic regulatory questions for various governmental agencies such as NRC (e.g., evaluation of exposures resulting from disposal of radioactive materials into sanitary sewer systems [Kennedy et al. 1991]).

- **Authorization Bases** – The GENII 1.485 system is used for determining the adequacy of operational requirements and emergency-response preparations, for safety-analysis reports (e.g., the Hanford 325 Building Safety Analysis Report), and safety bases for routine operations.

4.4 NRC's Integrated Multimedia Models and Systems

The NRC staff uses multimedia environmental assessment codes for reviewing license amendments for decommissioning and waste-disposal activities. Specifically, these include the Decontamination and Decommission (DandD), RESRAD, and MEPAS codes. The codes are used to review the licensees' conceptual models, evaluate various possible environmental pathways, and assess parameter inputs. The NRC staff reviews of the licensee's technical basis documents and their confirmatory analyses serve as a basis for license determinations.

For example, the NRC staff and its contractors have developed a methodology for calculating doses to demonstrate compliance with the radiological criteria for decommissioning and license termination as documented in NUREG-1549 "Decision Methods for Dose Assessment to Comply with Radiological Criteria for License Termination" (NRC 1998). The simplest method for calculating dose, generic screening, uses the DandD code and default parameters that the NRC developed for compliance screening calculations. The environmental pathways include both air and water, focusing on doses due to exposure, inhalation, and ingestion of residual radioactivity. Detailed information on the development and implementation of the dose-assessment methodology for decommissioning reviews is provided in the NUREG/CR-5512 technical series reports.

Specifically, NUREG/CR-5512, Volume 1, provides a description of the conservative scenarios and calculational approach for translating residual radioactivity to dose (Kennedy and Strenge 1992). Volume 2 is a User's guide for the DandD software (Wernig et al. 1999), which automates the dose calculations described in Volume 1. Volume 3 details the analysis used to define default parameter values for the Building Occupancy and Residential scenarios and the results of that analysis (Beyeler et al. 1999). Volume 4 documents the comparison of the models and assumptions used in the DandD Version 1.0, RESRAD Version 5.61, and RESRAD-Build Version 1.50 computer codes with respect to the residential farmer and industrial occupant scenarios provided in NUREG/CR-5512.[a]

To better understand the capabilities and uses of multimedia codes, the NRC staff convened a public "Workshop on Review of Dose Modeling Methods for Demonstrating Compliance with the Radiological Criteria for License Termination" at NRC Headquarters on November 13–14, 1997 (Nicholson and Parrot 1998). The workshop featured presentations and demonstrations by the developers of the multimedia environmental codes (i.e., MEPAS, DandD, RESRAD, FRAMES, and PRESTO) and facilitated discussions with them and the NRC staff, Agreement State regulators, licensees, EPA, DOE, and other stakeholders. Ongoing NRC-funded work includes modifications to the RESRAD and DandD codes to enable probabilistic applications within a risk-informed approach.

(a)   R. Haaker, T. Brown, and D. Updegraff. 1999. *Comparison of the Models and Assumptions used in the DandD 1.0, RESRAD 5.61, and RESRAD-Build 1.50 Computer Codes with Respect to the Residential Farmer and Industrial Occupant Scenarios Provided in NUREG/CR-5512 - Draft Report for Comment.* NUREG/CR-5512, Vol. 4, U.S. Nuclear Regulatory Commission, Washington, DC, October 1999.

4.4.1 Decontamination and Decommission

4.4.1.1 Purpose and General Attributes of DandD

DandD Version 2.1.0 performs probabilistic analyses of both scenarios and includes a sensitivity-analysis module that identifies parameters that have the greatest impact on the results of the dose assessment. The capability of importing soil and groundwater concentrations to be used as input for the dose assessment rather than relying on the models to simulate these values is available as an option for the residential scenario. This option enables assessment of dose from monitored data or allows the user to simulate these values with more complex models and evaluate the resulting dose with DandD. Context-sensitive online help is available to the user while running the DandD code as is much of the DandD supporting documentation. The DandD software and documentation are available at http://www.nrc.gov/RES/rescodes.htm.

4.4.1.2 Descriptive Summary of DandD

DandD is a tool developed by the NRC-RES to enable licensees to quickly and easily screen their site for compliance with the License Termination Rule. The DandD code implements the dose-assessment models developed in Volume 1 of NUREG/CR-5512 for multipathway exposure under a residential-farmer scenario and a building-occupancy scenario. DandD (Version 1) software was released in August of 1998, with the user's guide and parameter analysis documentation released in 1999. For compliance demonstration, the deterministic structure of Version 1 required a combination of default parameter values resulting in a degree of excess conservatism. In August 1999, the NRC-RES initiated the development of a probabilistic version of DandD (Version 2) that would not be encumbered by the restrictive default parameterization. Version 2 was released to the public in August of 2000 as a probabilistic tool for screening. Development is progressing on a revision for limited site-specific analysis.

DandD assists NRC licensees who must decontaminate lands and structures in determining the extent of decommissioning required to allow unrestricted release of their property. DandD Version 2.1.0 significantly enhances the capabilities of Version 1.0. In particular, Version 2.1.0 allows full probabilistic treatment of dose assessments, whereas Version 1.0 embodied constant default parameter values and only allowed deterministic analyses. DandD implements as an integrated model the methodology and information contained in NUREG/CR-5512, Volume 1, as well as the parameter analysis in NUREG/CR-5512, Volume 3, that established the probability distribution functions (pdfs) for all of the parameters associated with the scenarios, exposure pathways, and models embodied in DandD. Two scenarios are implemented in DandD: building occupancy and residential. The building-occupancy scenario relates volume and surface-contamination levels in existing buildings (presumably released following decommissioning for unrestricted commercial or light industrial use) to estimates of total effective dose equivalent (TEDE) received during a year of exposure with the conditions defined in the scenario. The exposure pathways for this scenario include external exposure, inhalation exposure, and secondary ingestion. The more complex and generalized residential scenario is meant to address sites with contamination in soils and groundwater. The residential scenario considers more exposure pathways; external exposure, inhalation, and the following ingestion pathways: drinking water, food grown from irrigation water, land-based food, soil, and fish. The types of land-based food considered are leafy vegetables, other vegetables, fruit, grain, beef, poultry, milk, and eggs. Three types of animal feeds are considered: forage, stored grain, and stored hay.

The draft report for comment, NUREG-1549, "Decision Methods for Dose Assessment to Comply with Radiological Criteria for License Termination," documents the use of a decision framework to implement a phased approach in conducting dose assessments. The decision framework can be used throughout the decommissioning and license-termination process for sites ranging from the more simple sites to the most complex or contaminated sites. The decision framework is based on the premise that screening dose assessments are performed with little site-specific information. An initial analysis using DandD and default DandD parameter distributions, along with a simple representation of contamination at the site, will produce generic dose assessments that are unlikely to be exceeded at real sites. The scenarios, models, and parameters in DandD were defined to be "reasonably conservative" such that they would not be "bounding" or unrealistic, while still generally overestimating rather than underestimating potential dose. The physical parameter distributions were defined to represent real conditions and expected variability across the United States. Behavioral and metabolic parameters were defined to represent the expected variability between individuals within the defined screening group (or generic critical group).

Licensees with relatively simple contamination patterns have a high assurance of complying with the decommissioning criteria in the NRC rule-making through the use of simple screening assessments. However, for licensees with more complex situations or who choose to perform more realistic analyses, the methodology ensures that as more site-specific information is incorporated (in later phases or iterations of the decision framework), the uncertainty is reduced (state of knowledge is increased), and the estimate of the resulting dose generally decreases. DandD Version 2.1.0 can be used to incorporate new knowledge based on site characterization that may lead to eliminating certain exposure pathways or reduced parameter uncertainty. DandD used in the context of the decision framework provides assurance (and helps optimize the decision) that obtaining additional site-specific information is worthwhile because it ensures that a more "realistic" dose assessment will not generally result in a dose higher than that estimated using screening.

The input parameter distributions for each scenario and exposure pathway were developed consistent with conducting screening dose assessments, increasing the likelihood of overestimating rather than underestimating potential dose. To accommodate site-specific conditions based on iterative use of the decision framework and new knowledge, the DandD software allows a simple, straightforward approach to modify scenario selection, exposure pathways, source profile, and many of the modeling parameters.

Finally, DandD Version 2.1.0 includes a sensitivity-analysis module that assists licensees and NRC users to identify those parameters in the screening analysis that have the greatest impact on the results of the dose assessment. Armed with this information and the guidance available in NUREG-1549, licensees are able to make informed decisions regarding the allocation of resources needed to gather site-specific information related to the sensitive parameters. When the cost and likelihood of success associated with acquiring this new knowledge are considered, licensees are better able to optimize the costs to acquire site data that allow more realistic dose assessments that, in turn, may lead to demonstrated and defensible compliance with the dose criteria for license termination. Context-sensitive online help is available to the user while running the DandD code as is much of the DandD supporting documentation. The DandD software and documentation are available at http://www.nrc.gov/RES/rescodes.htm.

4.4.1.3 Selected Applications of DandD

DandD is being applied by NRC licensees in the demonstration of compliance with the Radiological Criteria for License Termination (10 CFR 20 Subpart E). To allow unrestricted release of their property, NRC licensees may be allowed to use DandD to determine the extent of decontamination required to meet the criteria. DandD is useful as both a screening tool to demonstrate compliance for those sites that pose no risk to human health and safety using default probabilistic parameter distributions and generic scenarios, and as a tool for a range of site-specific analyses at sites that are conceptually consistent with the applicability of the code.

The NRC staff has also used both the MEPAS and RESRAD codes for conducting site-specific analyses. An example of where multimedia codes have been used in site-specific analysis is the West Valley Demonstration Project. For the West Valley site, the codes were used to evaluate EIS alternatives. Other licensing examples where multimedia codes are being used include the Sequoyah Fuels facility and the Parks Township decommissioning reviews. NUREG/CR-6566 documents the description of MEPAS Version 3.2 Modification funded by the NRC (Buck et al. 1997).

4.5 State's Integrated Multimedia Models and Systems

State government statutes and regulations are directly responsible for many monitoring and enforcement activities, which result in control of the flow of toxic chemicals into the environment. The legal structure and resulting programmatic function often constrain the use of multimedia and multi-source chemical fate and transport analysis. The current legal framework for government action needs to be analyzed for the potential efficiencies inherent in multimedia, analytic tools. The details of state decision making are based on rules established in the process agency interpretation of the language in the controlling federal statutes and the regional regulatory context. For example, remedial alternatives for waste sites are developed from a site analysis, which in part depends on the predicted transport of toxic chemicals to human receptors and an estimate of health risk. Many states have tailored superfund guidance specifically for regional landscape conditions, such as rainfall and general proximity of water bodies. However, property boundaries of the site in question often limit the scope of the investigation, and it is not extended to other sites in the immediate area to determine aggregate exposure and health effects. Air sources and deposition are not considered in managing hazardous site cases if they do not originate with the responsible party, and the contribution of land sources is not generally considered in point-source air-risk assessments.

The result of the single-media, one-source-at-a-time regulatory approach is that in areas with numerous sources side by side, it is possible for every source to be in compliance while the exposure resulting from all of them may exceed benchmark concentrations. There are some regulatory approaches, such as TMDLs and environmental justice initiatives, which are more likely candidates for multimedia analysis. TMDL determination inherently integrates multiple sources for the large land areas associated with watersheds. Environmental-justice evaluation calls for the summing of multiple sources of potential toxic chemical exposure to estimate community risk. Because both of these programs involve an analysis of sources that arise in multiple media, which must be summed, they are inherently more receptive to multimedia modeling methods than regulations driven by point source.

Sorting out the single-media modeling output as obtained from various regulatory programs so that aggregate or spatially or temporally resolved predicted media concentrations are available is probably impossible. This means that the relative importance or competing sources cannot be determined. A better approach would involve cross communicating single-media models or a comprehensive multimedia model used as the backbone for regulatory activities in all environmental media. Unconnected multimedia models applied to single-media sources can also cause problems. EPA'S OSWER combustor guidance and superfund guidance each move chemicals through multiple-media pathways, but by different algorithms. For example, the relationship between air and soil concentrations of the same chemical will be different in the different multimedia models. These contradictions do not become a noticeable problem until regulatory efforts start to overlap spatially. This is much more likely in densely industrial parts of the country. This is where chemical transport models that are trans-programmatic, multimedia, and multi source are most needed.

5.0 Software Attributes for Linking Models, Databases, and Frameworks

Prepared by G. Whelan and G.F. Laniak

The objective of the meeting was to convene a multi-agency group of exposure and risk modelers and assessors to investigate common protocols for the future design, implementation, and application of environmental models. The motivation for this workshop is the realization that with the increasing complexity of environmental assessments and decreasing funding, it is not plausible to expect one funding agency to have the required expertise. To move to a common protocol (or multiple protocols) on improving the communication linkage between disparate models, databases, and systems, it is important to describe the qualities (attributes) that software should contain to meet this lofty objective. These attributes represent the first and most important step to ensure that future software contains the qualities that allow it to communicate with other software. These attributes do not necessarily represent the qualities desired by every participant, as these attributes may, in fact, conflict with current software design, but current software design was not the point of the meeting. Based on these attributes, software can be designed, and specifications can be developed, to implement the design. A tentative list of attributes has been developed. The process of developing the attributes is described, and various groupings of the attributes are explored.

5.1 Process Procedure and Attribute Listing

Before the workshop, many of the participants were asked to help develop an initial list of software attributes, related to future multimedia modeling systems, from which a dialogue could be based. To help set the stage for developing a more refined list of attributes, and in an effort to ensure that the participants equally understand the meaning of each attribute, each of the attributes was reviewed before in-depth discussions in breakout sessions. Questions on the meaning of the attributes were fielded at this time, but questions on their validity were relegated to the breakout sessions.

Four attribute breakout sessions were established, and a facilitator was assigned to each session. The role of the facilitator was to (1) discuss the merits of each attribute, (2) keep the discussion on track and moving forward so all attributes were discussed, (3) prioritize the attributes both in importance and from a tactical (near-term) and strategic (long-term) point of view, and (4) summarize the findings of the group, including the issue with those that did not meet the consensus of the group. The intent of each group was to modify, delete, add, and prioritize attributes.

These attributes represent the qualities that the participants would expect future software to contain to facilitate communication between disparate models, databases, and systems. These attributes represent input from a number of organizations, are tentative, and require refinement, yet they represent a starting point for prioritizing and finalizing a more solidified list. The participants strived to be simple, but not simplistic, in identifying these attributes. Simple by definition means to be "easy to understand, deal with, and use." Simplistic means to "be absence of complexity and intricacy, lack good sense or intelligence, or be foolish."

Although not a result of this workshop, the results from each breakout session will eventually be used to propose universal designs for meeting those attributes. The design is not intended to be parochial or inflexible, but is intended to set the standard for allowing a number of different approaches to communicate. For example, if the attribute is to allow two models to seamlessly communicate, then the interface design between two models should be such that data should seamlessly pass from one model to the next, irrespective of scale or resolution (within reason) and should not be model dependent. A goal of the breakout session group was to identify attributes that help develop testable design criteria and to make suggestions on implementing the design, demonstrating its flexibility and transferability. Finally, each attribute was prioritized in importance, considering that the start of one recommendation may depend on the completion of another recommendation. Table 5.1 presents a summary and description of the attributes.

5.2 Grouping of Attributes

As noted earlier, a design is a comprehensive description of how a piece of software will function (i.e., how it will meet its attributes), and specifications are a detailed description of an interface to a computer program or set of subroutines such that another programmer could develop a program that would make proper use of the subroutines. In effect, the specifications describe the detail behind how one intends to implement the design. For example, if the attribute was to allow for the communication between two gridding systems (e.g., regular versus irregular), the design would define the conceptual model for mapping the two systems, and the specifications would allow a software engineer to write code to perform the mapping.

As part of the process to understand the inherent characteristics associated with the attributes, several crosscutting approaches were implemented to categorize and group the attributes. Because many of the attributes are complex in nature, they are inherently multi-dimensional and tend to be associated with multiple categories. Three different crosscutting approaches were independently discussed to inspect and categorize the attributes:

1. Grouping 1:   Model Connectivity, Information Architecture, Framework Connectivity, Web-based Access (including GIS), and System Functionality

2. Grouping 2:   Contract/Protocol, Framework/System Software Attributes, Network Attributes, Site/Scenario Conceptualization, Component Attributes, and Results Processing

3. Grouping 3: Input, Output, Process, Architecture

Table 5.1. Summary of the Attribute Characteristics

Attribute	Definition
1. Communication Protocol Between System, Models, and Databases	The interface protocol (contract) between the system and components (models and databases) needs to be defined in a precise manner. "Contract" describes the distribution of responsibility between the system and components, which allows for the linkage between models and databases. The intent of the system is to ensure the smooth transfer of information without placing unreasonable data-transfer requirements on the components. If a model or database meets linkage requirements, the system should allow them to communicate with other components. Communication protocol should a. represent a mutually agreed-upon contract between the system and those producing and consuming information (shared responsibility). b. be established so the system does not become too dependent on the models or databases linked within the system. The communication contract helps ensure that the system represents a conduit for communication, irrespective of the components involved in the communication process. Qualitatively, the system needs to maximize its role as a passive linkage facilitator. By maximizing its role as a conduit and coordinator of information, the system minimizes its dependency on which components comprise the system. This attribute refers to the distribution of responsibility for the transparent communication between models and between models and databases. For example, who is responsible for deciphering the information contained in a database: the model, system, or database? Who is responsible for understanding the "names" of the input parameters (which is different from the type of input) associated with a model: the model, system, or database? This attribute is testable when linkage protocols are established. c. be established to allow for the development of new interface protocols (contracts), where they are lacking, and provide guidance and techniques to preserve some degree of backward compatibility between versions of the software. d. allow for the capability to access information from multiple databases. It is also desirable to be able to pull the same type of information from a variety of similar databases, as a user option. For example, a user might want to conduct an ecological risk assessment using toxicity data from several different databases. This attribute should allow the framework to access any "linked" database and pull back the required information in a nearly seamless manner.

Table 5.1 (Contd)

Attribute	Definition
	e. allow for designs that appeal to multi-disciplinary groups by allowing multi-disciplinary models, databases, and frameworks to communicate.
	f. allow for changes and influence of COTS software, so the system grows as the state-of-the-art grows.
	g. allow the user to inspect the pedigree of the data to understand the quality of the data.
2. Data-Transfer Compatibility	The system design needs to strictly enforce data-transfer compatibility. Meta-data characteristics (name, type, cardinality, range, etc.) and pedigree of data need to be documented, where possible, realizing that the system cannot determine the correctness of the numbers. Meta-data characteristics should be checked through interface protocols (range checking of values, units checking, etc., if appropriate). Data-transfer compatibility can be ensured by a. clearly defining, accurately documenting, and strictly enforcing data-transfer specifications before implementing the system. Data that are transferred between models, but which are not associated with a naming protocol, need to be defined *a priori* through a data-transfer specification that is mutually agreed upon by the producing- and consuming-model types. The user is responsible for ensuring that a model's output meets the appropriate specifications that may only involve transfer of the values of the parameters and not their meta-data characteristics that have been accounted for in the documented specifications. This approach does not preclude the system from checking on the quality of the data (e.g., range checking). For example, the consuming surface-water model knows *a priori* the data format associated with a producing groundwater-model output. b. tracking the meta-data characteristics with the data itself. This approach uses a naming protocol that the system understands and which can be used to check the quality of the data that are being passed between models. Each model is privy to the parameters and nomenclature of other models through the system Application Program Interface (API).
3. Plug & Play and Intra-System Security Features	Plug & Play refers to the capability of the system to allow components to be added to or removed from the system in a relatively easy manner, allowing for transparent implementation of the component within the system. This feature should allow for the capability to include different classes of models if they currently do not exist in the system. For example, if a class of model (e.g., ecological) does not exist in the system, yet could use output from an existing class of model (e.g., surface water), the structure should be general enough to allow the communication with new or different models for future

Table 5.1 (Contd)

Attribute	Definition
	needs. With the Plug & Play attribute, a user should be able to select, connect, and apply/use a wide variety of models, modules, and databases in a relatively transparent and easily understood manner. Such an attribute provides ultimate flexibility, which is required for handling a broad spectrum of exposure- and risk-assessment problems. Directly related to Plug & Play is the capability of the system to allow the user to control components and how they interrelate to each other (intra-system security features). This feature helps prevent corruption of information transfer. Additionally, there is a need for lock & key features to prevent tampering with or overwriting files from previously conducted applications. Lock & key features refer to the capability to allow an organization to (1) fix the available models, CSM, and/or access to databases and (2) determine if the system as been inappropriately tampered with.
4. Legacy Codes	The system should allow for relatively easy incorporation of legacy codes. Models should retain their original ("legacy") form without requiring significant alteration. Linkage protocols should establish the distribution of responsibility for incorporating legacy models in a system. This may mean that system software may have to written to allow for and enforce an accepted protocol for connecting models and/or databases within the framework, such that it is not necessary to modify the framework or the model/databases when bringing new models/databases into the system. The system and its protocols should allow for easy integration of legacy models/databases into the system, such that these models can be "easily" structured (e.g., as modules) to communicate within this environment (make it as easy as possible for new models/databases/science to be integrated into the framework). The protocols that provide component linkage to the system need to be as easy to understand and apply as possible.
5. WEB-Based Connections	Allow for web-based (through Internet) connections for models and databases. Multiple options would be available here. Three situations are envisioned for models and databases alike: (1) run/access from a central host location, (2) run/access from multiple remote locations, and (3) download to the user's computer. The models and databases could be combined using one of these three in a number of different ways (e.g., 3x3=9). Web-enhanced features will allow access to web-based databases, access and application of models located at remote sites, and use of computing platforms at other locations.
6. Hardware Compatibility	The software system should be capable of communicating across a network of machines and be capable of running on a variety of machines (Windows 95 PC, Windows NT, Sun Workstation, Unix, etc.). Because Windows currently represents the largest client base, the system should at least have functionality to address Windows.

Table 5.1 (Contd)

Attribute	Definition
7. Software Compatibility	Allow for multiple computer languages (FORTRAN, C++, C, Java, even Prolog) to be used in developing components. The system needs to be accessible across multiple programming languages (FORTRAN 77, FORTRAN 90, C++, C, Java, even Prolog). This attribute is related to the Legacy Codes attribute, since models/databases may exist in a variety of languages and forms.
8. System User-Friendly Interface	Maintain a user-friendly interface for developing the CSM. The CSM should be intuitive and promote user-friendliness. An example, not necessarily a recommendation, of a user-friendly interface for constructing a CSM includes one that is an object-oriented, graphical user interface, where the user can click, drag, and connect icons (objects) to form a conceptual picture of the problem to be studied or modeled.
9. Component Ownership	Allow for ownership of components (models and databases) to be maintained by the modelers and database managers and not by the system. This attribute promotes the continued maintenance, upkeep, and QA/QC of legacy models and databases.
10. Feedback Between Models	Feedback refers to the capability for models to communicate on a real-time basis in space and time (two-way communication). For example, results from the model for benthic sediment contamination may be a function of results from a model for water-column contamination, which in turn is a function of the results of the model for benthic sediment contamination. Another example is when a vadose zone transfers sufficient quantities of water to cause mounding of the water table, which spatially and temporally modifies the aquifer flow field, and in turn impacts the vadose zone by reducing its spatial extent and modifying its flow field. This real-time feedback is an example of a closed loop. Feedback could be performed through the entire system by time step, or the feedback loop could be independent of the system and only a function of the individual models involved in communication, allowing for different time steps for different models. Typically, when feedback mechanisms are required, the models are linked outside the system and then imported as a linked module in the system.
11. Begin Assessment at Multiple Logical Entry Points	The system should be structured to allow the user to begin the analysis at any logical entry point to the system, in other words, to begin the assessment at any well-defined intermediate point in the assessment train. This functionality would allow the user to a. specify conditions that enhance and support the assessment process. For example, the user could vary the input boundary conditions to support model calibration to monitored data. b. use monitored data, as opposed to having to model and approximate a condition that is already well-defined. For example, there may be

Table 5.1 (Contd)

Attribute	Definition
	cases where observed exposure data exist and should be used, rather than running an exposure-assessment model.
	c. import information from models implemented outside of the system. The model results could be imported at specified locations most appropriate for their use. Many times a model has been previously run, producing output results that can be used in a follow-on assessment. In this case, it is unnecessary to link the model to the system, as only the data are needed.
12. Linkage to Other Frameworks	The system should be structured to allow for linkages to other frameworks. It may be advantageous to use another framework to conduct part of an analysis and then use output from that framework to continue the analysis in the user's framework. Linkages to other frameworks should be permitted in as nearly a seamless fashion as possible.
13. Communication Between Models of Differing Scale and Resolution	The system should be structured to allow for models of differing scale and resolution to communicate. Scale refers to the physical size and attributes of the problem (medium-specific, watershed, regional, global, etc.). Resolution refers to the temporal- and spatial-mesh resolution associated with the assessment (requirements associated with the transfer of data at medium interfaces [i.e., boundary conditions]), designated as low (e.g., structured-value), medium (e.g., analytical), and high (e.g., numerical). For example, an analytical model, using mass flux across an infinite plane should structure its output to be handled by another analytical model or numerical model containing a grid system. Another example is when two numerical models contain two different gridding systems with disparate time stepping. In each of these cases, a protocol needs to be established to allow the transfer of information with minimal loss of information such that mass is conserved. This does not exclude the possibility that multiple "sub" frameworks will be developed to address models with differing scales and resolutions. We need to distinguish between what a model calculates for its own numerical convergence/stability and what needs to be produced for consumption by other models.
14. Functionality of Modules in System	*Functionality of Modules in the System* refers to attributes that allow information to flow between modules (model types). Three attributes, considered important, include a. Multiple Sources – Contamination can originate from multiple sources, such as contaminated soil, water, stack emission, etc. There may also be multiple sources in the same medium. For example, known contaminant concentrations in soil may be available for several different locations where each location has a different pathway. One region may have several sources that contribute to the same receptor; as such, the system should have the capability to address the impacts and effects from all sources to obtain a

Table 5.1 (Contd)

Attribute	Definition
	holistic and systematic view of the impacts.
	b. Combining Output of Like Models – The system should allow the user to construct a CSM to combine the output of like modules. For example, if two models of the same type (groundwater, or air, or surface water, etc.) contribute contamination to the same location, then the effects of these contributions need to be addressed. Combining exposure to the same receptor from the same exposure routes (e.g., ingestion of contaminated water from a river and aquifer) represents another example.
	c. Secondary Sources – By definition, multimedia modeling takes a source emission and redistributes the contamination in the environment, resulting in additional areas of contamination. These new areas (or secondary sources) of contamination also represent potential sources from which contaminants can emanate. For example, a stack transfers contamination to the air, and contaminants are deposited through wet and dry deposition to the soil. Through the forces of leaching, volatilization, suspension, or runoff, contaminants may leave the soil and migrate into and through other media. The soil represents a secondary source, whereas the stack represents the primary source. The system needs to allow for the evaluation of secondary sources.
15. GIS Connectivity	Allow for GIS functionality. There may be a need to have access to a GIS. The software should be structured to allow access to GIS with the capability to import/export GIS information.
16. Visualization and Tabular Summation of Results	The system should be structured to provide for tabular summation of results. In some cases, it may be necessary to transfer results to special "form" reports for regulators, such as the Risk Assessment Guidelines for Superfund (RAGS). Complementing and expanding on the tabular summation of results are tools that allow the user to visualize the results. Visualization needs may vary from simple X-Y plots to more sophisticated 3-D color-coded plots. This functionality would include analysis and visualization of results generated by the system as well as data imported into the system. Visualization packages should be general and easily applied so the user can view all data, including model-input data.
17. Testable Components	Each component comprising the system should have the capability to stand alone and undergo testing, independent of the system. This functionality will enhance the capability to meet QA/QC requirements without unduly burdening the system or other models into being concurrently functional and operational. Testable components promote objective-oriented programming and corroborates the notion of independent objects.

Table 5.1 (Contd)

Attribute	Definition
18. Online Help	The software should include user-educational provisions. In addition to or connected with the profile information, the software should supply standardized descriptions associated with components. Style guides and/or HTML protocols for documentation should be used. Context-sensitive online help, possibly layered by expertise, should be supplied. As a secondary consideration, providing an "expert" system in the model-selection process, based on the models in the system, would help guide the user in not choosing the wrong model, which is different from providing guidance on choosing the"right" model (which may be impossible).
19. Mass Conservation	Mass should be conserved or accounted for throughout the system. The system is responsible for ensuring that the mass produced from one module is correctly transferred for consumption by the next downstream module. Mass balance within the module is the responsibility of the module, but differences between input and output within the module should be reported to the system.

These three groupings represent different conceptualization categorizations. For example, the first grouping represents the perspective of an environmental engineer, i.e., the mechanics of communication (Section 5.2): how to link models to models, models to databases, and frameworks to frameworks, and how to conceptualize and capture the problem. The second categorization represents the perspective of a systems engineer (Appendix E.1): system, network, and component protocols; problem definition; QA/QC; processing of results. The third represents the perspective of a software engineer (Appendix E.1): inputs, outputs, processes, and information architecture.

Even though these perspectives and categories are different, all of the attributes are captured, regardless of how the information is cross cut, illustrating the universality of the attributes and stressing the inclusive nature of the requirements. The workshop distributed the attributes into the first two groupings by category, but categorization of the attributes for the third grouping was only discussed during the workshop. Because the attributes can be categorized from different perspectives and to help ensure clarity, only the first set of groupings is presented in Chapter 5 (i.e., Grouping 1); Groupings 2 and 3 are presented in Appendices E.1 and E.2, respectively. By presenting Groupings 2 and 3 in Appendix E, this valuable information from the workshop is not lost and is available for future reference.

5.3 Model Connectivity, Information Architecture, Framework Connectivity, Web-Based Access, and System Functionality

Definitions of each category in this grouping are presented, and Table 5.2 presents the grouping of attributes by model connectivity, information architecture, framework connectivity, web-based access, and system functionality.

Table 5.2. Attribute Grouping by Model Connectivity, Database Connectivity, Framework Connectivity, Web-Based Access, and System Functionality

Attribute Grouping	Attribute Priority		
	High	Medium	Low
Model Connectivity	1, 3, 10, 13, 16, 17, 18, 19		
Database Connectivity	1, 2, 16		
Framework Connectivity	1, 12, 14, 19		
Web-Based Access	1, 5, 6, 15		
System Functionality	1, 2, 3, 4, 6, 7, 8, 9, 18, 19	10, 11, 14, 15, 16	

1. **Model Connectivity** – Model connectivity addresses the issues associated with ensuring the transparent linkage between models with the same and different scale and resolution (how models communicate with each other). Scale refers to the physical size and attributes of the problem (e.g., media-specific, watershed, regional, and global). Resolution refers to the temporal- and spacial-mesh resolution associated with the assessment (i.e., requirements associated with the transfer of data at media interfaces (boundary conditions), designated as low (structured-value), medium (analytical), and high (numerical). For example, an analytical model using mass flux across an infinite plane should structure its output to be handled by another analytical model or numerical model containing a grid system. Any design should be general enough and structured to ensure that mass is conserved and that the linkage handles most types of traditional models.

2. **Information Architecture** – Information architecture refers to the structure and protocol associated with accessing and transferring information between disparate databases and models. What are the most appropriate procedures for having a model access a disparate

database? Who has what responsibility? How does the model know that the data exist in the database or even how to access them? How does the database know what the model requires? This breakout session is probably the most important as the models cannot run without data, and more systems are attempting to use standardized databases in their assessments. For example, if a site-specific assessment does not contain enough information for the assessment to be completed, can the information be supplemented using a regional database (e.g., county soil surveys), or a national database (e.g., U.S. Department of Agriculture [USDA] soil type figures)?

3. **Framework Connectivity** – Framework connectivity addresses the issues associated with the transparent communication between systems (as opposed to models). In the past, a large number of single-medium models (e.g., river model) were developed. Since 1959, these single-medium models were being connected into more sophisticated frameworks that transparently linked these models together. Now, a fair number of frameworks have been developed and will continue to be developed. As models were linked together, frameworks will also eventually be linked together. This breakout session discusses the protocols for linking these systems in a transparent manner.

4. **Web-Based/GIS Access** – The fast-growing software arena is associated with the Internet. It is anticipated that researchers will eventually be accessing models and databases through the web. Multiple options associated with accessing models and databases and ensuring their connectivity are potentially available. For example, nine situations could be envisioned for connecting and running, where appropriate, models and databases: (1) run/access from a central host location, (2) run/access from multiple remote locations, and (3) download to the user's computer. The models and databases could be combined using one of these three in a number of different ways (i.e., 3x3=9). Web-enhanced features will allow access to web-based databases, access and application of models located at remote sites, and use of computing platforms at other locations. In addition, access to and utilization of GIS connectivity, dealing with spacial attributes, is also anticipated to be an important assessment resource in future waste-site analyses.

5. **System Functionality** – System functionality refers to the behavioral traits exhibited by and characteristics built into the system. For example, interface specifications to allow for the transfer of data between two models is a system property. Likewise, the structure that allows legacy codes to communicate is a system property; as long as the models follow linkage protocol, specified by the system, they can communicate.

6.0 Additional Ideas Generated from the March 2000 Workshop: Merging 3MRA and FRAMES-V1[a]

Prepared by G. Whelan, G.F. Laniak, M.A. Pelton, K.J. Castleton, M. Dortch, R. Cady,

D. Brown, J. Babendreier, and J.W. Buck

6.1 Summary

PNNL, under the guidance and direction of the EPA and DOE, developed the software technology system, titled Framework for Risk Analysis in Multimedia Environmental Systems (FRAMES). As a natural extension of the joint effort between DOE and EPA, EPA instructed PNNL to refine and extend FRAMES to build a technology software-modeling system capable of conducting a national assessment of exposure and risk due to contaminant releases from hazardous waste sites. This effort was to support the promulgation of rules associated with HWIR, using the 3MRA methodology.

The primary objective of this present effort is to design and implement enhancements to the FRAMES and 3MRA modeling technologies. FRAMES and 3MRA, while conceptually similar, are different in two fundamental ways. First, the manner in which data are managed in 3MRA is more advanced relative to FRAMES. Second, FRAMES was designed to facilitate site-specific assessments and thus has a user interface for collecting data from the user. The 3MRA system was designed to facilitate a national assessment and thus does not contain a site-specific user interface. The enhancements center on merging the best features of the existing 3MRA technology with the existing FRAMES technology and advancing the data-exchange protocols.

The first effort, as documented herein, is to develop and document attributes for a unified system, a unified CSM and a unified DEP. A CSM represents a simplified description of the environmental problem to be modeled. A DEP defines how data are transferred and exchanged between components (e.g., modules, databases, frameworks). Attributes are characteristics and behaviors that a piece of software must possess to function adequately for its intended purpose. The purpose of these attributes is to state those conditions that define the merger between FRAMES – Version 1 and the 3MRA software.

(a) From G. Whelan, M.A. Pelton, and J.W. Buck. 2001. *Merger Between 3MRA-HWIR and FRAMES-V1: Requirements.* PNNL-13453. Prepared for the Ecosystems Research Division, National Environmental Research Laboratory, Office of Research and Development, U.S. Environmental Protection Agency, Athens, Georgia, by Pacific Northwest National Laboratory, Richland, Washington.

6.2 Background

EPA is charged with developing, implementing, and enforcing regulations concerned with protecting human and ecological health from the myriad of chemical and non-chemical stressors imposed on the environment as a result of man's activities. DOE, in response to existing and emerging regulatory requirements for environmental protection, has developed a significant program for assessing exposure and risk at its facilities. In pursuing these activities, DOE and EPA share a common need to understand the environmental processes (physical, biological, and chemical) that collectively release, transform, and transport contaminants, resulting in exposure and finally a probability of deleterious health effects. At both EPA and DOE, computer models are key tools for organizing the knowledge of environmental science for application in the decision-making process.

The EPA and DOE have jointly pursued common interests related to environmental modeling. For example, in 1995, DOE's PNNL and EPA's Office of Air and Radiation in ORIA joined efforts to design and develop a prototype multimedia modeling system (Whelan et al. 1998a; 1998b; 1997). The unique aspect of this effort was to incorporate software modules representing individual steps of a risk assessment (source release of contaminants, fate and transport in various environmental media, exposure, etc.) within a software framework. The software framework was designed using "object-oriented design" and, as such, allowed for the decoupling of individual modules. This design greatly improved the ability of module developers (e.g., a modeler developing a new surface water module) to "plug" the new module into a full multimedia modeling system without the need to develop a complete modeling system. The product of this effort was FRAMES (Whelan et al. 1998a; 1998b; 1997). FRAMES allows a user to simulate contaminant-based exposure and risk in a multimedia environment at a single facility.

Concurrent to the development of FRAMES, DOE and the EPA'S ORD, Ecosystems Research Division in Athens, Georgia, also initiated a joint effort in 1995 to study existing technology and future needs of EPA and DOE related to multimedia/multipathway exposure and risk assessment. The initial focus of these early efforts was to conduct a benchmarking study involving three multimedia models: MEPAS, RESRAD, and MMSOILS. In 1995, the DOE/EPA modeling teams completed a Phase I report in which the operational characteristics of the three models were compared using a series of hypothetical contaminant-release problems (Whelan et al. 1999a, 1999b; Laniak et al. 1997; Mills et al. 1997; Cheng et al. 1995). This effort clearly demonstrated the significant similarity in design and approach to environmental modeling and the mutual benefit related to working together in future model-development activities. As a follow-on effort, an Inter-Agency Government (IAG) agreement was developed in 1996 in anticipation of a formal and long-term interagency effort to develop multimedia modeling tools and related technology to benefit both EPA and DOE. The initial focus of the IAG was to conduct a second phase of the benchmarking study. A new set of hypothetical problems extended the understanding developed in the original benchmarking work (Gnanapragasam et al. 2001; Whelan et al. 2000). A third follow-on study investigated the aspects associated with uncertainty analysis, using Monte Carlo simulation, between MMSOILS and the multimedia model PRESTO.

From 1998 through 2000, the joint effort between DOE and EPA was to extend and refine FRAMES to build a modeling system capable of conducting a national assessment of exposure and risk due to contaminant releases from hazardous waste sites (Laniak et al. 1999; Whelan and Laniak 1998a, 1998b). Coupled with the 3MRA methodology, EPA's OSW implemented a national assessment on HWIR. The 3MRA-HWIR system (also known as FRAMES-HWIR)[a] is being used to develop national exemption levels (contaminant concentration levels deemed *safe* in waste streams) that are part of a regulatory action to be published in the Federal Register (Lundgren and Whelan 1999).

In 1999-2000, the EPA's NERL responded to these needs by establishing specific R&D tasks to *integrate* all activities based on multimedia modeling, including the FRAMES-based efforts. The goal of this initiative is to design and implement, over the next decade, a MIMS that will facilitate future environmental assessments and related research. MIMS will contain a comprehensive set of modeling and assessment tools that can be applied to answer ever more complex questions of environmental impacts resulting from anthropogenic-based activities. MIMS is envisioned to address environmental impacts in a fully integrated fashion. Questions related to human exposure to multiple chemicals via numerous pathways and ecosystem sustainability will be at the core of future assessments. These questions will require modeling systems that simultaneously simulate the movement of chemicals through the environment, the impacts of land-use modifications, and population/community vulnerability within ecosystems. Further, because of the dramatic increase in the amount of information to be processed, MIMS will include state-of-the-art technologies for data visualization, transfer, and storage. In short, MIMS is focused on the next generation of holistic, systematic environmental modeling needs. MIMS guides current developmental efforts and represents the future of multimedia assessment systems. FRAMES, 3MRA, and other modeling systems, such as the technology being applied to EPA'S OW TMDL assessment, represent the current state-of-the-art in multimedia systems; they also represent deployed systems that are currently in use. EPA views FRAMES as (1) a technology for facilitating current site-based exposure and risk assessments and related modeling research and (2) a testing ground for investigating system-software concepts emerging from MIMS design discussions. It is intended that the move from FRAMES-based technologies (e.g., FRAMES and 3MRA) to MIMS-based technologies will be transparent to the user community. To achieve this, FRAMES will be used as a MIMS prototype and development environment.

Following the lead of DOE and EPA, USACE, ERDC-WES initiated the development of the ARAMS, based on the FRAMES technology, in calendar year 2000. The Army wanted a system that was compatible and consistent with the other Agencies, especially EPA. The Army is also cognizant of EPA's desire to develop a consistent and more universal approach to multimedia modeling. As such, ERDC-WES is cooperating with EPA in its development efforts by coordinating its activities with EPA. It is anticipated that ERDC-WES will follow protocols for software development that are consistent with current and future efforts by DOE and EPA. Although an explicit IAG between EPA and ERDC-WES has not been established for ARAMS, EPA has indicated that it recognizes ERDC-WES as a full partner in these activities. The intent is to continue and expand interagency working relationships among technical staff responsible for addressing multimedia-based issues. The

---

(a) For brevity, 3MRA, as applied to HWIR, will be noted as 3MRA in this chapter.

following benefits will accrue as a result of this joint effort between EPA, DOE, and ERDC-WES:

- The research will be driven by and thus enhance the regulatory process (i.e., development, implementation, and compliance) with respect to multimedia-based environmental concerns.

- Many specific technical issues must be resolved in addressing environmental concerns from the holistic multimedia perspective. This joint effort, by combining EPA and DOE expertise, will allow these modeling issues to be resolved in a more efficient, cost-effective, and scientifically defensible manner.

- The research will provide for a technically consistent linkage across the continuum of research, technology development, regulation development, compliance, and policy.

The development and modification activities associated with merging 3MRA, ARAMS, and FRAMES requires developing software and system attributes, design, and specifications. The attributes, which are outlined in Chapter 5, formed the basis for developing attributes associated with the merging of 3MRA and FRAMES, yet compatible with ARAMS. After multiple meetings during 2000 and 2001 and as a direct result of the March 2000 workshop's efforts, EPA, NRC, DoD, and PNNL clarified and slightly modified the attributes in Chapter 5 to meet the specific needs associated with the software-merging process. The functionality of the merged system will be incrementally developed, recognizing that the basic system structure governs future modifications and updates. Activities associated with developing a merged system have been divided into near-term and far-term. The attributes listed herein address near-term requirements. These attributes are presented in the following section.

6.3 Attributes Associated with the Merging of 3MRA and FRAMES-V1

Before presenting the attributes associated with the merged system, certain terms that are specific only to the merged system are defined.

6.3.1 Definitions

- **Database Owner Tool (DOT)** – support software that allows the database owner to map the information in the database to the FRAMES Data DICtionary (DIC) files. The DOT database holds the developed extraction plans (mappings), database schema, and the schema of the DIC. The DOT has already been developed and represents system (universal) software.

- **Data Extraction Tool (DET)** – extracts the data from the designated database and returns it to the DCE through the Hypertext Transfer Protocol (http). When invoked by the DCE, the DET goes out to the DOT database, retrieves the desired extraction plan from the DOT database, extracts the appropriate data through a Structured Query Language (SQL) server, and returns it to the DCE. The DCE then stores these data on the local drive in a designated file for eventual consumption by module icons (and their underlying models) connected to the dataset icon. The DET has already been developed and represents system (universal) software.

- **Database Client Editor (DCE)** – invokes the DET with an http request for data from the associated DIC. The DCE is a user interface that can view and edit the data. Each dataset icon Subgroup is associated with one DIC. The DCE is DIC specific, whereas the DIC essentially defines a dataset type (e.g., Database Class • Ecological Group • Eco Benchmarks Subgroup, whereas the Environmental Residue-Effects Database (ERED) would represent a database in this database Subgroup or type). The DCE retrieves the association between the DIC (e.g., Eco Benchmarks), database (e.g., ERED), and the DET URL from the command line options passed in, whereas the command line explains the association between the DIC, database, and DET URL. The data-set-icon-type DESCRIPTION (DES) file holds the associations that are passed to the DCE through the command line when invoked by FRAMES. The DES file will be created by the DOT after dataset mapping is complete. To date, a DCE has been developed for Eco Benchmarks and represents system (universal) software. No other DCEs have been developed.

- **FRAMES Server** – stores the system DICs and available database list with the associated DIC mappings. For every database -DIC mapping, there will be a DES file that the system DCE can use to connect to and retrieve data from the database. This software has not yet been developed.

- **Global Database** – represents a database that can be accessed by any module in the system.

- **Module** – consists of a model, pre- and post-processors, and MUI and represents a choice under an icon.

6.3.2 Unified System Considerations

Attributes for a Unified Conceptual Site Model (UCSM) and a Unified Data Exchange Protocol (UDEP) cannot be developed without considering attributes associated with the overall structure of the merged system. For example, the attributes for linking disparate models, and disparate models to disparate databases, need to be consistent with the attributes for the UCSM and UDEP. GIS connectivity, sensitivity/uncertainty, visualization of output, and system mass balance also need to be considered and compatible within the system. Transferring data and metadata requires a systematic, holistic approach that transcends the CSM and is compatible with a UDEP. This section summarizes the attributes associated with system functionality, recognizing that an attribute may fit into a number of attribute categories. The merged system shall

1. operate on a PC with Microsoft NT, WIN98, or Win2000 platforms with a minimum of 128-MB RAM Pentium or equivalent, and 1-GB free disk space

2. support Borland C^{++} Builder Version 5.0, Microsoft Visual C^{++} Version 5.0, Lahey FORTRAN-90 Version 4.0, and Fujitsu Visual FORTRAN-90 Version 5.0 compilers

3. allow for the functionality of entering the system at specified locations (e.g., import a file, user-specified information)

4. be capable of essentially implementing the 3MRA analysis by integrating 3MRA modules and processors into the new design so they essentially function in a manner consistent with the original 3MRA implementation

5. be capable of having functional compatibility, not necessarily backward compatibility, with 3MRA and FRAMES-V1. Functional compatibility means that a 3MRA problem can be implemented in the new system to produce the same results. By being compatible with FRAMES-V1, the merged system would have the capability of developing a CSM to implement a site-specific 3MRA analysis.

6. allow for superposing like information using a system-support *plus operator*

7. allow for secondary sources without feedback to the source

8. be capable of documenting assumptions, surrogate names (aliases), changes in imported data from database, and version-control changes in pop-up or sticky notes, summary file(s), and/or a report generator

9. provide standardized reports and plots, initially supplying the current plotting capabilities of FRAMES-V1 and tabularized results associated with the FRAMES report generator and EPA RAGS Part D

10. contain a print feature

11. allow for multistage Sensitivity/Uncertainty (S/U) (i.e., S/U inside an S/U)

12. include online help for system-only components

13. include security features for accessing and implementing the merged system

14. incorporate lock and key features that allow a user to lock a CSM picture, available models, and/or both

15. allow for models to run on different platforms (e.g., remote computing)

16. be configured to handle multiple directories for scenario and module files (like 3MRA)

17. provide for unit conversions

18. include confidence intervals on cumulative probabilities.

6.3.3 Unified Conceptual Site Model Considerations

Consistent with the system considerations, the UCSM represents a protocol for conceptualizing a physical area (i.e., contaminated site) for the purpose of simulating source release, fate and transport through multiple media, and human and ecological exposure/risk. The UCSM will have the site-specific plug & play functionality of FRAMES and the operational attributes of implementing national assessments of 3MRA. It is anticipated that the user will eventually be able to address the national assessment by (1) directly populating the databases that drive it, as is currently done in 3MRA, or (2) constructing the databases site-by-site, using the FRAMES drag & drop features. The starting point for discussions will be the existing protocols and CSMs for FRAMES and 3MRA. This section summarizes the attributes associated with the unified conceptual site model and graphical user interface, recognizing that an attribute may fit into a number of attribute categories. The merged system shall

19. develop the CSM using Visual Basic, possibly American National Standards Institute (ANSI) C or Java

20. allow for tiered icons (primary and secondary icons)

21. allow for the icon pallette to expand to include additional icons, when appropriate

22. divide the icon palate by Domain, Class, Group, and SubGroup

23. include a standard set of icons (including a standard set of database icons) that encompasses those associated with FRAMES-V1 and 3MRA

24. allow for the functionality to add new module icons, if desired

25. be capable of developing a CSM with the drag & drop features from FRAMES-Version 1 (FRAMES-V1)

26. allow for multiple sources.

6.3.4 Unified Data Exchange Protocol Considerations

Consistent with system and UCSM attributes, the UDEP will maintain the site-specific plug & play functionality of FRAMES and the operational attributes of implementing national assessments of 3MRA. It is anticipated that the user will eventually be able to address the national assessment by (1) directly populating the databases that drive it, as is currently done in 3MRA, or (2) constructing the databases site-by-site, using the FRAMES drag & drop features. The UDEP shall include both a *low-level* protocol that addresses the exchange of individual data items from one system component to another and a *high-level* protocol that ensures the capability to share components of the current technologies. The current technologies include Global Input Data (GID) and Primary Communication Data File (PCDF) file structures within FRAMES and the Site Simulation Files (SSF), Global Results Files (GRF), and DIC file structures within 3MRA. The starting point for discussions will be the existing data-exchange protocols for FRAMES and 3MRA. It is anticipated that attributes will be included to address access to, extraction from, and exchange of data from databases that may or may not reside on the host machine. This section provides a summary of the attributes associated with the unified data exchange protocol and database connectivity, recognizing that an attribute may fit into a number of attribute categories. The merged system shall

27. provide for different database types (e.g., chemical, ecological benchmarks, and human-health benchmarks) by representing each type by separate icons on the icon palette. The database icons should have the same linkage functionality as other icons associated with the system (allow for one database to supply information to a downstream database).

28. provide a DCE for system chemical- and lifeform-specific databases, which allows for identifying surrogates for (i.e., aliasing of) chemicals and/or lifeforms associated with each database type. The DCE allows for modification of imported database parameters when data are retrieved from the database (e.g., override human-health toxicity benchmarks and ecological Toxicity Reference Values [TRVs], from Integrated Risk Information System [IRIS] and Environmental Residue-Effects Database [ERED] databases, respectively).

29. map database information and parameters when the database is first invoked

30. design the capability to link outside frameworks to the system by allowing for icons on the icon pallette to describe those outside frameworks. The framework icons should eventually have the same linkage functionality as other icons associated with the system

31. allow a set of databases to supply information to a receiving module, establishing data priority on the same information

32. account for GIS connectivity

33. design for time-varying CSM, but not implement the design for a time-varying CSM

34. design the input/output and spacial/temporal linkage datafile specifications in the system through an API, which accounts for units and range checking and parameter attributes

35. allow for the linkage of disparate models (e.g., analytical and numerical) in space and time

36. account for at least three dimensions for spatially based parameters with a design that would allow for the incorporation of time as a fourth dimension

37. include, as part of module specifications, mass entering/leaving a module, where appropriate

38. allow viewing of data attributes for modules chosen to represent icons in the CSM before implementing the CSM

39. provide for global databases by way of master lists that can be updated from the FRAMES data server.

7.0 References

10 CFR 20, Subpart E,"Radiological Criteria for License Termination," July 1997.

Beyeler, W., W.A. Hareland, F.A. Duran, T.J. Brown, E. Kalinina, D.P. Gallegos, and P.A. Davis, "Residual Radioactive Contamination from Decommissioning: Parameter Analysis," NUREG/CR-5512, Vol. 3, Draft for Comment, U.S. Nuclear Regulatory Commission, October 1999.

Booch, G., *Object-Oriented Analysis and Design with Applications,* The Benjamin/Cummings Publishing Company, Inc., Redwood City, California, 1993.

Boulton, W.J., M. Lepage, W. Jiang, *Application of the Models-3 Framework to a Canadian Urban Airshed.* Institute for Chemical Process and Environmental Technology (ICPET), National Research Council (NRC) Canada, Ottawa, Ontario, Canada, 1999.

Buck, J.W., M.S. Peffers, and S.T. Hwang, "Preliminary Recommendations on the Design of the Characterization Program for the Hanford Site Single-Shell Tanks — A System Analysis," PNL-7573, Vol. 2, Pacific Northwest Laboratory, Richland, Washington, 1991.

Buck, J.W., G.M. Gelston, and W.T. Farris, "Scoring Methods and Results for Qualitative Evaluation of Public Health Impacts from the Hanford High-Level Waste Tanks," PNNL-10725, Pacific Northwest Laboratory, Richland, Washington, 1995.

Buck, J.W, D.L. Strenge, B.L. Hoopes, J.P. McDonald, K.J. Castleton, M.A. Pelton, and G.M. Gelston, "Description of Multimedia Environmental Pollutant Assessment System (MEPAS) Version 3.2 Modification for the Nuclear Regulatory Commission," NUREG/CR-6566, U.S. Nuclear Regulatory Commission, Washington, DC, November 1997.

Cheng, J.J., J.G. Droppo, E.R. Faillace, E.K. Gnanapragasam, R. Johns, G. Laniak, C. Lew, W. Mills, L. Owen, D.L. Strenge, J.F. Sutherland, G. Whelan, and C. Yu (in alphabetical order), "Benchmarking Three Multimedia Models: Description, Analysis, and Comparison of RESRAD, MMSOILS, and MEPAS," DOE/ORO-2033, U.S. Environmental Protection Agency, Athens, Georgia, and U.S. Department of Energy, Washington, DC, 1995.

Coats, C., "The EDSS/Models-3 I/O API," available at http://www.iceis.mcnc.org/EDSS/ioapi/, 1998.

Congressional Commission on Risk Assessment and Risk Management (CRARM), *Commission on Risk Assessment and Risk Management. Risk Assessment and Risk Management in Regulatory Decision-Making*, Final report, Volume 2, Washington, DC, 1997.

DOE, see U.S. Department of Energy.

Droppo, J.G., Jr., J.W. Buck, J.S. Wilbur, D.L. Strenge, and M.D. Freshley, "Single-Shell Constituent Rankings for Use in Preparing Waste Characterization Plans," PNL-7572, Pacific Northwest Laboratory, Richland, Washington, 1991.

EPA, see U.S. Environmental Protection Agency.

Gelston, G.M., M.F. Jarvis, R. Von Berg, and B.R. Warren, "Development and Application of Unit Risk Factor Methodology: Nevada Test Site," PNL-10608, Pacific Northwest Laboratory, Richland, Washington, 1995.

Gnanapragasam, E.K., C. Yu, G. Whelan, W.B. Mills, J.P. McDonald, C.S. Lew, C.Y. Hung, and D. Hoffmeyer, "Comparison of Multimedia Model Predictions for a Contaminant Plume Migration Scenario," *J. Contam Hydrol.* (accepted), 2001.

Hartz, K.E., and G. Whelan, "MEPAS and RAAS Methodologies as Integrated into the RI/EA/FS Process, in *Proceedings of the 9th National Conference: Superfund '88*, Hazardous Materials Control Research Institute, Silver Spring, Maryland, November 28–30, pp. 295–299, 1988.

Hyman, M. and L. Bagaasen, "Select a Site Cleanup Technology," *Chem. Eng. Prog*, pp. 22–43, August 1997.

Kennedy, W.E., M.A. Parkhurst, R.L. Aaberg, K.C. Rhoads, R.L. Hill, and J.B. Martin, "Evaluation of Exposure Pathways to Man From Disposal of Radioactive Material Into Sanitary Sewer Systems," NUREG/CR-5814, U.S. Nuclear Regulatory Commission, Washington, DC, 1991.

Kennedy, W. and D. Strenge, "Residual Radioactive Contamination from Decommissioning: A Technical Basis for Translating Contamination Levels to Annual Total Effective Dose Equivalent" NUREG/CR-5512, Vol. 1, U.S. Nuclear Regulatory Commission, Washington, DC, 1992.

Kossik, R., and I. Miller, *GoldSim User's Guide*, Golder Associates Inc., downloadable at http://www.goldsim.com/software, 2001a.

Kossik, R. and I. Miller, *GoldSim Contaminant Transport Module User's Guide*, Golder Associates Inc., downloadable at http://www.goldsim.com/software, 2001b.

Laniak, G.F., J.G. Droppo, Jr., E.R. Faillace, E.K. Gnanapragasam, W.B. Mills, D.L. Strenge, G. Whelan, and C. Yu (alphabetical order), "An Overview of a Multimedia Benchmarking Analysis for Three Risk Assessment Models: RESRAD, MMSOILS, and MEPAS," *Risk Analysis*, 17(2):203–214, 1997.

Laniak, G.F., K.J. Castleton, and G. Whelan, "An Overview of a National Multimedia, Multipathway, and Multireceptor Risk Assessment Technology Development," in *Proceedings of the 1999 Annual Meeting for Society of Risk Analysis*, Atlanta, Georgia, December 5–8, 1999.

Leigh, C.D., B.M. Thompson, J.E. Campbell, D.E. Longsine, R.A. Kennedy, and B.A. Napier, "User's Guide for GENII-S: A Code for Statistical and Deterministic Simulations of Radiation Doses to Humans from Radionuclides in the Environment," SAND91-0561A, Sandia National Laboratories, Albuquerque, New Mexico, 1992.

Lundgren, R.E. and G. Whelan, "FRAMES-HWIR Technology Software System -- System Overview," PNNL-11914, Vol. 1, Pacific Northwest National Laboratory, Richland, Washington, 1999.

Mills, W.B., J.J. Cheng, J.G. Droppo, Jr., E.R. Faillace, E.K. Gnanapragasam, R.A. Johns, G.F. Laniak, C.S. Lew, D.L. Strenge, J.F. Sutherland, G. Whelan, and C. Yu (alphabetical order), "Multimedia Benchmarking Analysis for Three Risk Assessment Models: RESRAD, MMSOILS, and MEPAS," *Risk Analysis*, 17(2):187–202, 1997.

Napier, B.A., R.A. Peloquin, D.L. Strenge, and J.V. Ramsdell, "GENII – The Hanford Environmental Radiation Dosimetry Software System," PNL-6584, Vols. 1–3, Pacific Northwest Laboratory, Richland, Washington, 1988.

Nicholson, T.J., and J. Parrot, "Proceedings of the Workshop on Review of Dose Modeling Methods for Demonstration of Compliance with the Radiological Criteria for License Termination," NUREG/CP-0163, U.S. Nuclear Regulatory Commission, Washington, DC, 1998.

NRC, see U.S. Nuclear Regulatory Commission.

Onishi, Y., S.B. Yabusaki, C.R. Cole, W.E. Davis, and G. Whelan, *Multimedia Contaminant Environmental Exposure Assessment (MCEEA) Methodology for Coal-Fired Power Plants, Volumes I and II*, prepared for RAND Corporation by Battelle, Pacific Northwest Laboratories, Richland, Washington, 1982.

Onishi, Y., A.R. Olsen, M.A. Parkhurst, and G. Whelan, "Computer-Based Environmental Exposure and Risk Assessment Methodology for Hazardous Materials," *J. Haz. Mat.*, 10:389–417, 1985.

Pacific Northwest National Laboratory (PNL), "ReOpt Version 3.1," PNL-7840, Rev. 3, Pacific Northwest Laboratory, Richland, Washington, 1995.

Pacific Northwest National Laboratory (PNL), "RAAS Version 1.1," PNL-8751, Rev. 3, Pacific Northwest Laboratory, Richland, Washington, 1996.

Poston, T.M., R.W. Hanf, and R.L. Dirkes, "Hanford Site Environmental Report for Calendar Year 1999," PNNL-13230, Pacific Northwest National Laboratory, Richland, Washington, 2000.

Schreckhise, R.G., K. Rhoads, J.S. Davis, B.A. Napier, and J.V. Ramsdell, "Recommended Environmental Dose Calculation Methods and Hanford-Specific Parameters," PNL-3777, Rev. 2, Pacific Northwest Laboratory, Richland, Washington, 1993.

U.S. Department of Energy (DOE), "Decommissioning of Eight Surplus Production Reactors at the Hanford Site, Richland, Washington," DOE/EIS-0119D, Washington, DC, 1989.

U.S. Department of Energy (DOE), "Hanford Remedial Action Draft Environmental Impact Statement," DOE/DEIS-0222, Vols. 1 and 2, Richland, Washington, 1994.

U.S. Department of Energy (DOE), "Hanford Site Spent Nuclear Fuel Management Program," DOE/EIS-0203-F, prepared for the U.S. Department of Energy by Pacific Northwest Laboratory, Richland, Washington, 1995a.

U.S. Department of Energy (DOE), "Management of Spent Nuclear Fuels from the K-Basins at the Hanford Site, Richland, Washington – Environmental Impact Statement," DOE/EIS-0245D, prepared for the U.S. Department of Energy by Pacific Northwest Laboratory, Richland, Washington, 1995b.

U.S. Department of Energy (DOE), "Medical Isotopes Production Project: Molybdenum-99 and Related Isotopes – Environmental Impact Statement," DOE/EIS-0249-D, prepared for the U.S. Department of Energy by Pacific Northwest Laboratory, Richland, Washington, 1995c.

U.S. Department of Energy (DOE), "Medical Isotopes Production Project: Molybdenum-99 and Related Isotopes," DOE/EIS-0249F, Washington, DC, 1996.

U.S. Department of Energy and Washington State Department of Ecology (DOE/DOE), "Tank Waste Remediation System, Hanford Site, Richland, Washington, Final Environmental Impact Statement," DOE/EIS-0189, Richland, Washington, 1996.

U.S. Environmental Protection Agency (EPA), "Users Manual for the Human Exposure Model (HEM)," EPA-540/5-86-001, Office of Air Quality Planning and Standards, Research Triangle Park, North Carolina, 1986.

U.S. Environmental Protection Agency (EPA), "Mercury Study Report to Congress," EPA-452/R-97-005, Volumes I–VIII, Office of Air Quality Planning and Standards, Research Triangle Park, North Carolina, 1997.

U.S. Environmental Protection Agency (EPA), "Study of Hazardous Air Pollutants from Electric Utility Steam Generating Units," Final Report to Congress, EPA 453/R-989-004a, Office of Air Quality Planning and Standards, Research Triangle Park, North Carolina, 1998.

U.S. Environmental Protection Agency (EPA), "Residual Risk Report to Congress," EPA-453/R-99-001, Office of Air Quality Planning and Standards, Research Triangle Park, North Carolina, 1999a.

U.S. Environmental Protection Agency (EPA), "Methodology for Assessing Health Risks Associated with Multiple Pathways of Exposure to Combustor Emissions," EPA 600/R-97/137, Office of Research and Development, National Center for Environmental Assessment, Washington, DC, 1999b.

U.S. Environmental Protection Agency, "National Air Toxics Program: The Integrated Urban Strategy," 64 FR 38705–38740, July 19, 1999.

U.S. Nuclear Regulatory Commission (NRC), *Science and Judgment in Risk Assessment,* National Research Council, National Academy Press, Washington, DC, 1994.

U.S. Nuclear Regulatory Commission (NRC), *Building A Foundation for Sound Environmental Decisions,* National Research Council, National Academy Press, Washington, DC, 1997.

U.S. Nuclear Regulatory Commission (NRC), "Decision Methods for Dose Assessment to Comply with Radiological Criteria for License Termination," NUREG-1549, Washington, DC, 1998.

Wernig, M.A., A.M. Tomasi, and C.D. Updegraff, "Residual Radioactive Contamination from Decommissioning: User's Manual," Draft Report, NUREG/CR-5512, Vol. 2, U.S. Nuclear Regulatory Commission, Washington, DC, May 1999.

Whelan, G., D.L. Strenge, J.G. Droppo, Jr., and B.L. Steelman, "Overview of the Remedial Action Priority System (RAPS)," in *Pollutants in a Multimedia Environment,* Y. Cohen (ed.)., Plenum Press, New York, pp. 191–227, 1986.

Whelan, G., D.L. Strenge, J.G. Droppo, Jr., B.L. Steelman, and J.W. Buck, "The Remedial Action Priority System (RAPS): Mathematical Formulations," DOE/RL/87-09, PNL-6200, prepared for the U.S. Department of Energy's Office of Environment, Safety, and Environment by Pacific Northwest Laboratory, Richland, Washington, 1987.

Whelan, G., J.W. Buck, D.L. Strenge, J.G. Droppo, Jr., B.L. Hoopes, and R.J. Aiken, "An Overview of the Multimedia Assessment Methodology MEPAS," *Haz. Waste Haz. Mat.* 9(2):191–208, 1992.

Whelan, G., J.P. McDonald, and C. Sato, "Environmental Consequences to Water Resources From Alternatives of Managing Spent Nuclear Fuels at Hanford," PNL-10053, prepared for the U.S. Department of Energy by Pacific Northwest Laboratory, Richland, Washington, 1994.

Whelan, G., J.W. Buck, A. Nazarali, and K.J. Castleton, "Assessing Multiple Waste Sites Using Decision-Support Tools," in *Application of Geographic Information Systems in Hydrology and Water Resources Management*, K. Kovar and H. P. Nachtnebel (eds.), International Association of Hydrological Sciences, Publication No. 235, IAHS Press, Institute of Hydrology, Wallingford, Oxfordshire, OX10 8BB, United Kingdom, pp. 373–381, 1996.

Whelan, G., K.J. Castleton, J.W. Buck, G.M. Gelston, B.L. Hoopes, M.A. Pelton, D.L. Strenge, and R.N. Kickert, "Concepts of a Framework for Risk Analysis in Multimedia Environmental System (FRAMES)," PNNL-11748, Pacific Northwest National Laboratory, Richland, Washington, 1997.

Whelan, G. and G.F. Laniak, "A Risk-Based Approach for a National Assessment," in *Risk-Based Corrective Action and Brownfields Restorations*, C.H. Benson, J.N. Meegoda, R.B. Gilbert, and S.P. Clemence (eds.), in *Geotechnical Special Publication Number 82*, American Society of Civil Engineers, Reston, Virginia, pp. 55–74, 1998.

Whelan, G., J.W. Buck, B.L. Hoopes, K.J. Castleton, M.A. Pelton, and G.M. Gelston, "Concepts Associated with a Framework for Risk Analysis in Multimedia Environmental Systems," in *Proceedings of the American Nuclear Society – Topical Meeting on Risk-Based Performance Assessment and Decision Making*, PNNL-SA-30475, American Nuclear Society, La Grange Park, Illinois, 1998a.

Whelan, G., J.W. Buck, K.J. Castleton, B.L. Hoopes, M.A. Pelton, J.P. McDonald, G.M. Gelston, and R.Y. Taira, "Framework for Risk Analysis in Multimedia Environmental Systems (FRAMES)," T.J. Nicholson and J.D. Parrot (eds), in *Proceedings on the Workshop on Review of Dose Modeling Methods for Demonstration of Compliance with the Radiological Criteria for License*, NUREG/CP-0163, U.S. Nuclear Regulatory Commission, Washington, DC, 1998b.

Whelan, G., J.P. McDonald, E.K. Gnanapragasam, G.F. Laniak, C.S. Lew, W.B. Mills, and C. Yu, "Benchmarking of the Vadose-Zone Module Associated with Three Risk Assessment Models: RESRAD, MMSOILS, and MEPAS," *Environ. Engineer. Sci.*, 16(1):93–103, 1999a.

Whelan, G., J.P. McDonald, E.K. Gnanapragasam, G.F. Laniak, C.S. Lew, W.B. Mills, and C. Yu, "Benchmarking of the Saturated-Zone Module Associated with Three Risk Assessment Models: RESRAD, MMSOILS, and MEPAS," *Environ. Engineer. Sci.*, 16(1):67–80, 1999b.

Whelan, G., J.P. McDonald, E.K. Gnanapragasam, C.Y. Hung, C.S. Lew, W.B. Mils, and C. Yu, "Source-Term Development for a Contaminant Plume for Use by Multimedia Risk Assessment Models," *J. Contam. Hydrol.*, 41:205–223, 2000.

Yu, C., A.J. Zielen, J.J. Cheng, Y.C. Yuan, L.G. Jones, D.J. LePoire, Y.Y. Wang, C.O. Loureiro, E. Gnanapragasam, E. Faillace, A. Wallo III, W.A. Williams, and H. Peterson, *Manual for Implementing Residual Radioactive Material Guidelines Using RESRAD,* Version 5.0, ANL/EAD/LD-2, Argonne National Laboratory, Argonne, Illinois, 1993.

APPENDIX A

AGENDA

APPENDIX A

AGENDA

ENVIRONMENTAL SOFTWARE SYSTEMS

COMPATIBILITY AND LINKAGE WORKSHOP

NRC HEADQUARTERS TRAINING FACILITY

March 7-9, 2000

Day 1: Tuesday, March 7, 2000		
Day's Objective:	Establish the protocols for lines of communication and compatibility between databases, models, and systems. In other words, where are we ultimately going and with what constraints.	
8:00 - 8:30am	Sign-In at NRC	Two White Flint Building/Front Desk
8:45 - 9:00	Welcome	NRC-NMSS & RES Staff Management
9:00 - 9:30	Meeting Objectives/Agenda Review	Tom Nicholson, NRC-RES
9:30 - 9:45	Participant Introductions	Jack Parrot, NRC-NMSS
9:45 - 10:00	NRC Objectives	Ralph Cady, NRC-RES
10:00 - 10:15	DOE - FRAMES Objectives	Paul Beam, DOE-EM
10:15 - 10:30	EPA - Models 2000 Objectives	Dave Brown, EPA-ORD
10:30 - 10:45	EPA-Athens Objectives	Dave Brown/Gerry Laniak, EPA-ORD
10:45 - 11:00	BREAK	
11:00 - 11:15	PNNL Objectives	John Buck, PNNL
11:15 - 11:30	EPA-OSW Objectives	Zubair Saleem, EPA-OSW
11:30 - 11:45	EPA-ORIA Objectives	Chris Nelson/Dale Hoffmeyer, EPA-ORIA
11.45 - 12:00	ERDC-WES-ARAMS Objectives	Mark Dortch, ERDC-WES (ARAMS)
12:00 - 12:15 pm	ERDC-WES-LMS Objectives	Jeff Holland, ERDC-WES (LMS)
12:15 - 1:15	LUNCH	
1:15 - 1:30	RESRAD Dose Modeling Objectives	Charley Yu, ANL
1:30 - 1:45	ORNL (EPA-OAQPS) Objectives	Brad Lyon, ORNL
1:45 - 2:00	Model Transparency (BIOMOVS/BIOMASS)	Chris McKenney, NRC
2:00 - 2:15	Golder Objectives	Ian Miller, Golder
2:15 - 3:00	Summarizing Initial List of Overall Attributes	Mark Dortch, ERDC-WES
3:00 - 3:30	BREAK	
3:30 - 4:50	Attribute Breakout Sessions, T-3B15	Tom Nicholson, NRC-RES
	1. Attribute Breakout Group 1, T-3B39	Gerry Laniak, Facilitator
	2. Attribute Breakout Group 2, T-3C	Zubair Saleem, Facilitator
	3. Attribute Breakout Group 3, T-3C2	Mark Dortch, Facilitator
	4. Attribute Breakout Group 4, T-3B15	Jeff Holland, Facilitator
4:50 - 5:00	Review Day's Activities/ Announcements	Tom Nicholson, NRC-RES

Day 2: Wednesday, March 8, 2000		
Day's Objective:	Review of where we are in the development cycle, as it relates to the attributes. Review design and specifications for information compatibility and transferability between listed attributes and currently available models and frameworks.	
8:00 - 8:15am	Sign-In at NRC	
8:15 - 8:30	Review Day's Agenda/Announcements, T-3B15	Tom Nicholson, NRC
8:30 - 9:00	Summary of Attributes	Facilitators
9:10 - 12:00	15-min presentations of current methodologies [focusing on how their approaches were designed to address the LISTED ATTRIBUTES and which attributes they were designed to address]	
9:10 - 9:25	Models 2000	Dave Brown, EPA-ORD
9:30 - 9:45	MIMS	Karl Castleton, EPA-ORD
9:50 - 10:05	FRAMES	John Buck, PNNL
10:10 -10:25	BREAK	
10:30 - 10:45	3MRA	Zubair Saleem, EPA-OSW
10:50 - 11:05	GENII-2	Chris Nelson/Dale Hoffmeyer, EPA-ORIA
11:10 - 11:25	ARAMS	Mark Dortch, ERDC-WES (ARAMS)
11:30 - 11:45	LMS	Jeff Holland, ERDC-WES (LMS)
11:50 - 12:05pm	RESRAD	Charley Yu, ANL
12:05 - 1:05	LUNCH	
1:10 - 1:25	DandD	Ralph Cady, NRC-RES
1:30 - 1:45	TRIM	Brad Lyon, ORNL
1:50 - 2:05	GoldSim	Ian Miller, Golder
2:10 - 4:45	Summary of Attribute Breakout Sessions, T-3B15	ALL
4:45 - 5:00	Review Day's Activities/Announcements	Tom Nicholson, NRC-RES

Day 3: Thursday, March 9, 2000		
Day's Objective:	Finalize attributes and provide a hands-on demonstration of software that may meet some of the attributes.	
8:00 - 8:15am	Sign-In at NRC	
8:15 - 8:30	Review Day's Agenda/Announcements, T-3B15	Tom Nicholson, NRC-RES
8:30 - 11:00	Summary of Attribute Breakout Sessions, T-3B15	ALL
11:00 - 12:00	Overall Summary of Breakout Findings	Gerry Laniak, EPA-ORD
12:00 - 1:00pm	LUNCH	
1:00 - 4:00	Hands-On Demonstration of Software, Room T-3B39	

A.2

APPENDIX B
PARTICIPANTS

APPENDIX B

PARTICIPANTS

ENVIRONMENTAL SOFTWARE SYSTEMS
COMPATIBILITY AND LINKAGE WORKSHOP
NRC HEADQUARTERS TRAINING FACILITY
March 7-9, 2000

Boby Abu-Eid
Mail Stop T-7F3
U.S. NRC
Washington, DC 20555
BAE@NRC.GOV

Paul Beam
Environmental Management
U.S. Department of Energy, Headquarters
19901 Germantown Road
Germantown, MD 20874-1290
301-903-8133
paul.beam@em.doe.gov

Dave Brown
U.S. EPA National Exposure Research Laboratory/ORD
Ecosystems Research Division
960 College Station Road
Athens, GA 30605-2720
706-355-8300
brown.dave@epa.gov

John Buck
Mail Stop K6-80
P.O. Box 999
Pacific Northwest National Laboratory
Richland, WA 99352
509-376-5442
john.w.buck@pnl.gov

Ralph E. Cady
Mail Stop T-9F31
U.S. NRC
Washington, DC 20555
REC2@NRC.GOV

Lansana Coulibaly, PhD
New Jersey Institute of Technology
Civil and Environmental Engineering Dept.
Newark, NJ 07102
973-596-6077
lxc7629@njit.edu

Pat Deliman
CEERD-ES-Q
U.S. Army Corps of Engineers
Engineer Research and Development Center
3909 Halls Ferry Road
Viscksburg, MS 39180-6199
601-634-3623
DELIMAP@wes.army.mil

Mark Dortch
U.S. Army Corps of Engineers
Engineer Research and Development Center
ATTN: CEERD-EP-W
3909 Halls Ferry Road
Vicksburg, MS 39180-6199
601-634-3517
dortchm@wes.army.mil

James Droppo
Mail Stop K6-80
P.O. Box 999
Pacific Northwest National Laboratory
Richland, WA 99352
509-376-7652
James.Droppo@PNL.GOV

John Greeves
Mail Stop T-7J8
U.S. NRC
Washington, DC 20555
JTG1@NRC.GOV

Bob Hazen
New Jersey Department of Environmental Protection
401 E. State Street
7th Floor, East Wing
P.O. Box 402
Trenton, NJ 08625-0402
609-292-8294
bhazen@dep.state.nj.us

Dale A. Hoffmeyer
Mail Code 6608J
U.S. EPA Headquarters
Ariel Rios Building
1200 Pennsylvania Avenue, N. W.
Washington, DC 20460U.S. EPA
202-564-9228
Hoffmeyer.Dale@epamail.epa.gov

Jeffrey P. Holland
CEERD-CHL
U.S. Army Corps of Engineers
Engineer Research and Development Center
3909 Halls Ferry Road
Vicksburg, MS 39180-6199
601-634-2644
HOLLANJ@wes.army.mil

Cheng-Yeng Hung
Mail Code 6608J
U.S. EPA Headquarters
Ariel Rios Building
1200 Pennsylvania Avenue, N. W.
Washington, DC 20460
202-564-9204
hung.cheng-yeng@epa.gov

Stephen Kroner
Mail Code 5307W
U.S. EPA Headquarters
Ariel Rios Building
1200 Pennsylvania Avenue, N. W.
Washington, DC 20460
703-308-0468
kroner.stephen@epa.gov

Gerry Laniak
U.S. EPA National Exposure Research Laboratory/ORD
Ecosystems Research Division
960 College Station Road
Athens, GA 30605-2720
706-355-8316
Laniak.Gerry@epamail.epa.gov

Donald Loomis
Sandford Cohen & Associates
1355 Beverly Road, Suite 250
McLean, VA
703-893-6600
dloomis@scainc.com

Brad Lyon
1060 Commerce Park
Oak Ridge National Laboratory
Oak Ridge, TN 37831
865-241-2649
LYONBF@ORNL.GOV

C. Thomas Marr, Jr.
Program Manager, Information Sciences & Engineering
Pacific Northwest National Laboratory
Mail Stop K7-63
P.O. Box 999
Richland, WA 99352
(509) 375-4349
tom.marr@pnl.gov

Christopher McKenney
Mail Stop T-7F3
U.S. NRC
Washington, DC 20555
CAM1@NRC.GOV

Ian S. Miller
GoldSim Consulting Group
Golder Associates Inc.
18300 NE Union Hill Road, Suite 200
Redmond, WA 98052
425-883-0777
software@goldsim.com

Tin Mo
Mail Stop T-9F31
U.S. NRC
Washington, DC 20555
TXM@NRC.GOV

Sam Nalluswami
Mail Stop T-7F27
U.S. NRC
Washington, DC 20555
SMN@NRC.GOV

Christopher B. Nelson
Mail Code 6608J
USEPA Headquarters
Ariel Rios Building
1200 Pennsylvania Avenue, N. W.
Washington, DC 20460
202-564-9209
nelson.chris@epa.gov

Thomas J. Nicholson
Mail Stop T-9F31
U.S. NRC
Washington, DC 20555
301-415-6268
TJN@NRC.GOV

Jack Parrot
Mail Stop T-8F37
U.S. NRC
Washington, DC 20555
301-415-6700
JDP1@NRC.GOV

Mitch Pelton
Mail Stop K6-80
P.O. Box 999
Pacific Northwest National Laboratory
Richland, WA 99352
509-376-1824
mitch.pelton@pnl.gov

George E. Powers
Mail Stop T-9F31
U.S. NRC
Washington, DC 20555
GEP@NRC.GOV

Carlos E. Ruiz
CEERD-ES-Q
U.S. Army Corps of Engineers
Engineer Research and Development Center
3909 Halls Ferry Road
Vicksburg, MS 39180-6199
601-634-3784
ruizc@wes.army.mil

Zubair Saleem
Mail Code 5307W
U.S. EPA Headquarters
Ariel Rios Building
1200 Pennsylvania Avenue, N. W.
Washington, DC 20460
703-308-0467
saleem.zubair@epa.gov

Cheryl Trottier
Chief, Radiation Protection, Environmental Risk and Waste Management Branch
U.S. NRC
Mail Stop T-3F31
Washington, DC 20555
301-415-7000
Cat1@nrc.gov

Gene Whelan
Mail Stop K9-36
P.O. Box 999
Pacific Northwest National Laboratory
Richland, WA 99352
509-372-6098
Gene.Whelan@pnl.gov

Tony Wolbarst
Mail Stop 6608J
U.S. EPA Headquarters
Ariel Rios Building
1200 Pennsylvania Avenue, N. W.
Washington, DC 20460
202-564-9392
Wolbarst.Anthony@epamail.epa.gov

Charlie Yu
Argonne National Laboratory (East)
9700 South Cass Avenue
Argonne, IL 60439
630-252-5589
CYU@ANL.GOV

Supporters of the Workshop who were unable to attend

Justin Babendreier
U.S. EPA National Exposure Research Laboratory/ORD
Ecosystems Research Division
960 College Station Road
Athens, GA 30605-2720
706-355-8344
Babendreiere.Justin@epamail.epa.gov

King Boynton
Water Environment Research Foundation
601 Wythe Street
Alexandria, Virginia 22314
703-684-2470
kboynton@werf.org

David Cozzie
Mail Code 5307W
U.S. EPA Headquarters
Ariel Rios Building
1200 Pennsylvania Avenue, N. W.
Washington, DC 20460
703-308-0479
cozzie.david@epa.gov

James Danna
Mail Stop T-7F3
U.S. NRC
Washington, DC 20555
JGD@NRC.GOV

Barnes Johnson
Mail Code 5307W
U.S. EPA Headquarters
Ariel Rios Building
1200 Pennsylvania Avenue, N. W.
Washington, DC 20460
703-308-8881
johnson.barnes@epa.gov

Deirdre L Murphy
Mail Code MD-13
U.S. EPA Mailroom
Research Triangle Park, NC 27711
919-541-0729
Murphy.Deirdre@epamail.epa.gov

William R. Ott
Deputy Branch Chief
Radiation Protection, Environmental Risk, Waste Management Branch
Mail Stop T-9F31 T-7F3
U.S. NRC
Washington, DC 20555
WRO1@NRC.GOV

Mark Thaggard
Mail Stop T-7F3
U.S. NRC
Washington, DC 20555
MXT3@NRC.GOV

James Thomas
Mail Stop T-7F27
U.S. NRC
Washington, DC 20555
JDT@NRC.GOV

APPENDIX C

RELATED WEB SITES

APPENDIX C

RELATED WEB SITES

ARAMS

ARAMS information can be found at:

http://www.wes.army.mil/el/arams/

ERDC

ERDC Modeling systems information can be found at two locations:

http://www.denix.osd.mil/LMS

http://chl.wes.army.mil/software

FRAMES

Information on FRAMES can be found at:

FRAMES software information - http://mepas.pnl.gov:2080/earth/

FRAMES software installation - http://mepas.pnl.gov:2080/frames/

FRAMES Data File Specifications -

GENII-2

Information on GENII-2 can be found at:

GENII-2 software information - http://mepas.pnl.gov:2080/earth/

GENII-2 software installation - http://mepas.pnl.gov:2080/frames/

GoldSim

Information on the GoldSim model can be found at:

http://www.goldsim.com

HWIR

HWIR Rule information can be found at:

http://www.epa.gov/epaoswer/hazwaste/id/hwirwste/risk.htm

LMS

Information on LMS can be found at:

www.denix.osd.mil/LMS/

MEPAS

Information on MEPAS can be found at:

MEPAS software information - http://mepas.pnl.gov:2080/earth/

MEPAS software installation - http://mepas.pnl.gov:2080/frames/

Models 2000 and Models 2001

Information on Models 2000 and Models 2001 can be found at:

www.epa.gov/ordntrnt/ORD/CREM

RCRA Docket

Society of Environmental Toxicology and Chemistry (SETAC) Meeting information can be found at:

http://www.setac.org

TRIM

TRIM draft technical support documents and status report for TRIM can be found at:

http://www.epa.gov/ttn/uatw/urban/trim/trimpg.htm

WMS

WMA general information can be found at:

http://chl.wes.army.mil/software/wms/

3MRA Model

3MRA general information can be found at: http://www.epa.gov/CEAM

APPENDIX D

SUMMARY OF COMMENTS OF PARTICIPANTS

APPENDIX D

SUMMARY OF COMMENTS OF PARTICIPANTS

Bob Hazen

New Jersey Department of Environmental Protection

401 E. State Street

7th Floor, East Wing

P.O. Box 402

Trenton, NJ 08625-0402

609-292-8294

bhazen@dep.state.nj.us

This workshop presents perhaps the best hope for interagency collaboration in a discipline noted for complexity and fragmentation. It was clear from the presentations that enormous efficiencies are within reach for such a group which demonstrated quite astonishing unity of purpose. It did seem, however, that most work has been with large complicated high priority sites with dispersion as the notable modeling paradigm. The need for the reconciliation of effects from thousands of smaller sources within a radius of tens of kilometers in a densely populated area as occurs in New Jersey does not appear to be typical or well-studied on a national scale.

APPENDIX E

ALTERNATIVE APPROACHES

TO GROUPING ATTRIBUTES

APPENDIX E

ALTERNATIVE APPROACHES TO GROUPING ATTRIBUTES

E.1 Contract/Protocol, Framework/System Software Attributes, Network Attributes, Site/Scenario Conceptualization, Component Attributes, and Results Processing

A second grouping of attributes was also suggested during the workshop and is represented by Contract/Protocol, Framework/System Software Attributes, Network Attributes, Problem (Site/Scenario) Conceptualization, Component Attributes, and Results Processing. The definitions of these terms are presented as follows.

1. **Contract/Protocol** – Contract/Protocol represents those attributes that address linkage specifications for transparent communication between disparate models and databases.

2. **Framework/System Software Attributes** – Framework/System Software Attributes refer to system attributes that help the user maintain quality assessments and control the options that are used in the assessment. Features allowing the user to pick and choose models, entering the assessment at specified points and locking CSMs or models for the assessment, represent examples in this category. Range checking and internal-security features also represent examples of attributes associated with this category.

3. **Network Attributes** – This category refers to those attributes that address web-based Internet connections.

4. **Problem (Site/Scenario) Conceptualization** – This category refers to those attributes that enhance the ability of the user to develop and accurately characterize the problem conceptualization (e.g., CSM).

5. **Component Attributes** – Component attributes refer to those attributes that are specific to the components that populate the system, including issues related to ownership, type of model (e.g., air, aquifer, surface water), being independently testable, having online help, and ensuring internal conservation of mass.

6. **Results Processing** – Results processing refers to those attributes that support the analysis and compilation of results, including spacial relationships and visual and tabular summaries.

Table E.1 presents the grouping of attributes by Contract/Protocol, Framework/System Software Attributes, Network Attributes, Problem (Site/Scenario) Conceptualization, Component Attributes, and Results Processing.

E.2 Input, Output, Process, and Architecture

A third grouping of attributes was also suggested during the workshop and is represented by Input, Output, Processes, and Architecture. The definitions of these terms are presented as follows.

1. **Input** – Input is information or data transferred or to be transferred from a producing medium to a consuming medium. Any data/information that are required to process a model (output from one model may be input to another). Input can be provided through a variety of structures, including database format (flat or relational), manual entry, and parameter files. Data owner and trustee responsibilities need to be defined. In addition, the system needs to provide access to data, regardless of location (local or remote machines) for review/evaluation purposes, and to provide the ability to extract data, regardless of location (local or remote machines). The system should allow or provide the ability to extract a complete database or selected records, tables, or fields, by either a query or FTP. Also, the resulting data structures could be flat or relational.

2. **Output** – Output is computer results (e.g., answers to mathematical problems; statistical, analytical, or accounting figures; or production schedules) or information transferred from a producing medium to a consuming medium and represents any data/information that are provided as a result of processing a model (output from one model may be input to another). Output can be provided in different structures, including databases (flat and relational) or graphical. Where appropriate, the system should allow use of existing output formats and provide optional outputs in report, tabular, graphic, and advanced visualization formats.

3. **Process** – Process is a generic term that may include compute, assemble, compile, interpret, and generate. Herein, it refers to the transformation of input data into output data. A process may include the ability to (1) transform data using calculations or formulas (e.g., creating a new field based on values in one or more existing fields or changing values of a field based on calculations), (2) resolve temporal and spatial scaling issues, (3) extract either on demand or via a scheduling process, (4) evaluate intermediate files during a process, (5) determine storage and processing requirements before the process begins, (6) allow the generation of "scenarios" that can be saved and reused, and (7) create test scenarios

4. **Architecture** – Architecture is comprised of four components, described as follows:

    a. Data Architecture – Data Architecture refers to the data structure required to perform activities, including data-administration requirements. There should be two levels of MetaData: required and optional. MetaData should be kept with data as it is extracted, and new MetaData will be generated as new data are created. The system should provide the ability to evaluate data against predefined criteria.

    b. Hardware Architecture – Hardware Architecture refers to the physical environment (servers, routers, cables, etc.) required to perform activities. The system should be web-based, not browser or platform specific, and processing should be allowed on single or multiple machines, local or remote. The system should also be designed to be flexible and expandable.

c. Security Architecture – Security Architecture refers to security processes and rules, including remote access, password rotation, and anti-virus procedures. The system should provide appropriate levels of security, and this security management should be distributed, not centralized..

d. Software Architecture – Software Architecture refers to the software environment required to perform activities. The User Interface should be easy to use and intuitive, and, where appropriate, the application should be allowed to use the existing User Interface.

Because the workshop did not group the attributes according to Input, Output, Process, and Architecture, a summary table is not provided.

Table E.1. Attribute Grouping by Contract/Protocol, Framework/System Software Attributes, Network Attributes, Site/Scenario Conceptualization, Component Attributes, and Results Processing

Attribute Grouping	Attribute Priority		
	High	Medium	Low
Contract/Protocol	1, 2, 13	10	
Framework/System Software Attributes	1, 2, 3, 6, 18, 19	4, 11	7
Network Attributes	5, 6	12	
Problem (Site/Scenario) Conceptualization	8, 15	11, 14	
Component Attributes	3, 9, 17, 18, 19	10, 13	
Results Processing	16	15	

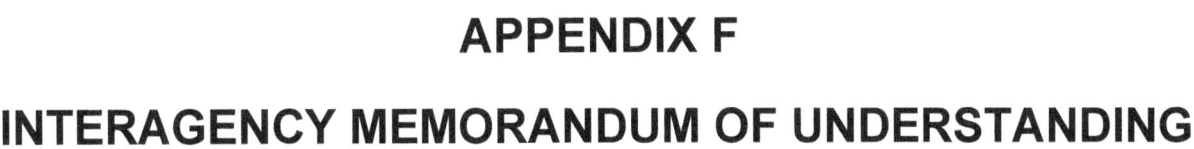

APPENDIX F

INTERAGENCY MEMORANDUM OF UNDERSTANDING

APPENDIX F

INTERAGENCY MEMORANDUM OF UNDERSTANDING

THE UNITED STATES NUCLEAR REGULATORY COMMISSION
OFFICE OF NUCLEAR REGULATORY RESEARCH

THE UNITED STATES ENVIRONMENTAL PROTECTION AGENCY
OFFICE OF RESEARCH AND DEVELOPMENT
NATIONAL EXPOSURE RESEARCH LABORATORY

THE UNITED STATES ARMY CORPS OF ENGINEERS
ENGINEER RESEARCH AND DEVELOPMENT CENTER

THE UNITED STATES DEPARTMENT OF ENERGY
OFFICE OF SCIENCE AND TECHNOLOGY

THE UNITED STATES DEPARTMENT OF THE INTERIOR
U.S. GEOLOGICAL SURVEY

THE UNITED STATES DEPARTMENT OF AGRICULTURE
AGRICULTURAL RESEARCH SERVICE

I. Purpose

a. The purpose of this Memorandum of Understanding (MOU) is to establish a framework for facilitating cooperation and coordination among the United States Nuclear Regulatory Commission (NRC), Office of Nuclear Regulatory Research (RES); the United States Environmental Protection Agency (EPA), Office of Research and Development (ORD), National Exposure Research Laboratory; the United States Army Corps of Engineers (COE), Engineer Research and Development Center (ERDC); the United States Department of Energy (DOE), Office of Science and Technology; the United States Department of the Interior (DOI), U.S. Geological Survey (USGS); and the United States Department of

Agriculture (USDA), Agricultural Research Service (ARS) in research and development (R&D) of multimedia environmental models, software and related databases, including development, enhancements, applications and assessments of site-specific, generic, and process-oriented multimedia environmental models as they pertain to human and environmental health risk assessment. This MOU does not include agency work directly in support of licensing activities.

b. This MOU is intended to provide a mechanism for the cooperating Federal Agencies to pursue a common technology in multimedia environmental modeling with a shared scientific basis.

c. This MOU is intended to reduce redundancies and improve the common technology through exchange and comparisons of multimedia environmental models, software and related databases. By entering into this MOU, the cooperating Federal Agencies seek mutual benefit from their respective R&D programs related to multimedia environmental model development and enhancement activities, and to ensure effective exchange of information between their technical staff and contractors. The R&D programs referred to here include development and field applications of a wide variety of software modules, data processing tools, and uncertainty assessment approaches for understanding and predicting contaminant transport processes including the impact of chemical and non-chemical stressors on human and ecological health.

d. This MOU focuses on exchange of information related to multimedia environmental modeling tools and supporting scientific information for environmental risk assessments, protocols for establishing linkages between disparate databases and models, and development and use of a common model-data framework.

e. This MOU is intended to facilitate the establishment of working partnerships among the cooperating Federal Agencies' technical staff and designated contractors in order to enhance productivity and mutual benefit through collaboration on mutually-defined research studies such as the development of a common model-data framework.

II. Authorities

Nothing in this MOU will be construed to alter the statutory authorities and/or limitations of the cooperating Federal Agencies. The authorities for NRC to enter into this MOU are the Section 205 of the Energy Reorganization Act of 1975 (42USC5845) and the Economy Act of 1932 as amended (31USC1535). The authorities for DOE to enter into this MOU are sections 646(a) (42USC7256(a)) and 102(11) and (13) (42USC7112(11) and (13)) of the Department of Energy Organization Act of 1977. USDA, ARS enters into this MOU under the authority of 7 U.S.C. 3318(b). The legal authority for the other cooperating Federal Agencies to enter into this MOU is the Economy Act of 1932, as amended (31USC1535). This MOU does not supersede or void existing memoranda of understanding or other agreements among the cooperating Federal Agencies.

III. Responsibilities

The cooperating Federal Agencies agree to:

a. Designate staff-level points of contact for the cooperating Federal Agencies. For the NRC, the staff-level point of contact will be at NRC Headquarters, within the Radiation Protection, Environmental Risk and Waste Management Branch, Office of Nuclear Regulatory Research. For EPA, the staff-level point of contact will be the Chief, Regulatory Support Branch, Ecosystems Research Division, National Exposure Research Laboratory. For the COE, the staff-level point of contact will be the Chief, Water Quality and Contaminant Modeling Branch, Environmental Processes and Engineering Division, Environmental Laboratory. For the DOE, the staff-level point of contact will be with the Office of Science and Technology or the Office of Integration and Disposition. For the USGS, the staff-level point of contact will be with the National Research Program, Branch of Regional Research, Central Region. For the ARS, the staff-level point of contact will be the Associate Deputy Administrator, Natural Resources and Sustainable Agricultural Systems, National Program Staff, Beltsville, Maryland.

The designated points of contact will promote technical coordination, identify joint R&D programs of mutual interest for the Federal Agencies and funding for such programs, and will assist in arranging for supplemental interagency agreements for R&D projects on multimedia environmental models, software and related databases at appropriate sites and laboratories.

The designated points of contact also will facilitate the coordination and exchange of R&D data and technical information related to environmental risk assessment modeling among the cooperating Federal Agencies. They will represent their individual agency's R&D programs and facilities conducting R&D as it pertains to modeling of human and ecological health impacts.

The designated points of contact will be responsible only for research activities and technical information exchanges identified in this MOU and not those directly in support of licensing activities.

The cooperating Federal Agencies further agree that the designated points of contact will serve as members of a Steering Committee. Alternates may be designated by the Federal Agencies to represent specific technical interests. The purpose of this committee will be to coordinate joint research efforts under this MOU. The committee will initially meet in the Washington, DC area within four months of the effective date of this MOU, and thereafter at least annually at various locations (or through teleconferencing) as determined by the Steering Committee members. Participation in technical working groups established by the Steering Committee, and at technical meetings called by the Steering Committee, will be determined by the cooperating Federal Agencies.

b. Cooperate in selected R&D programs of the other cooperating Federal Agencies by providing resources, information and technical expertise for review (outside of the conventional research peer review process) or consultation in areas of multimedia environmental model development, enhancements, applications, and assessments subject to program priorities and budget constraints.

c. Support the exchange of technical information through data bases, information systems, clearinghouses, conferences, workshops, activities for developing a common model-data framework, collaboration on scientific projects supporting the modeling framework, and other means pertaining to multimedia model development, enhancements and applications focusing on environmental risk assessments, subject to program priorities and budget constraints.

d. Support approved research at selected sites by providing services, facilities, utilities and other supporting resources as appropriate and subject to program priorities and budget constraints. Details of such support will be more specifically identified in supplemental interagency agreements (IAG's) prepared in accordance with applicable laws and regulations, and subject to the availability of funds.

Specific IAG's among the cooperating Federal Agencies will be developed pursuant to this MOU whenever appropriate to define specific undertakings. Such IAG's may provide for cooperative projects, or other efforts deemed appropriate, subject to applicable laws and regulations pertaining to the respective agencies and the availability of funds.

Details of support for specific cooperative work including funding, project plans, designation of cooperative work, and details of program management and execution will be contained in the IAG's. The cooperating Federal Agencies' program officials will communicate directly with one another during the planning and execution of these IAG's.

IV. Administration

It is the policy of the cooperating Federal Agencies to make the results of the R&D work contemplated by this MOU available to the public consistent with applicable security and other regulations.

a. Technology transfer: The participating Federal Agencies will establish procedures for sharing multimedia environmental models, software, related databases and supporting scientific information with the other cooperating Federal Agencies. Since the Federal Agencies have specific statutory patent policies regarding inventions funded in whole or in part by the Federal Government, the patent policies of the agency conducting the work shall apply to agreements executed between the parties to the MOU as well as to contracts they are under where such agreements or contracts are funded in whole or in part by the cooperating Federal Agencies. The cooperating Federal Agencies shall resolve any conflicts in their patent polices on a case-by-case basis when they enter into implementing IAG's. In all other circumstances it is agreed that the governing patent and data policies will be determined in accordance with the policy of the sponsoring agency.

b. Information release: All data and information originating from these cooperative research studies will be published and made available to the public as authorized by law through the cooperating Federal Agencies' public information and publishing procedures.   This information and data will not be disseminated to anyone, except the cooperating Federal Agencies, until such time as it is made available to the public by the originating Federal Agency. The parties will ensure that their contractors will disseminate such information in accordance with this agreement and the cooperating Federal Agencies' procedures.

The cooperating Federal Agencies agree to share any press releases or other public affairs information related to joint efforts or projects for review and concurrence prior to release.

c. Financial policy: It is recognized that the cooperating Federal Agencies have specific statutory requirements and limitations that dictate their financial policies. Therefore, the cooperating Federal Agencies agree to consider and specifically to address the financial policies to be applied to each project under the authority of this MOU as a term of the individual IAG's detailing each such R&D project.

d. Program funding: Although this MOU is neither a fiscal nor a funds obligating document, each cooperating Federal Agency will seek to ensure sufficient funding to carry out projects that are mutually agreed upon as a result of this MOU. The details of the levels of funding to be furnished one agency by the others will be developed in specific IAG's. The cooperating Federal Agencies will provide mutual support in budget justifications to the Office of Management and Budget and in hearings before Congress with respect to programs on which they collaborate. The cooperating Federal Agencies agree that this MOU does not involve the exchange of funds, and further that any correlated IAG's entered by two or more of the cooperating Agencies will be subject to the availability of funds appropriated by the Congress for such purposes.

e. Public information coordination: Subject to the Freedom of Information Act (5USC552), decisions on disclosure of information to the public regarding projects and programs implemented under this MOU will be made following consultation among the cooperating Federal Agencies' representatives.

f. Amendment and termination: This MOU may be modified and amended by written agreement among the cooperating Federal Agencies or terminated by mutual written agreement of the Federal Agencies. An individual agency may withdraw from the MOU upon 90-day written notice to the other agencies.[a]

g. Quality assurance: An important goal of the MOU and subsequent IAG's is high- quality research and modeling products. The cooperating Federal Agencies commit to following their established quality assurance (QA) and quality control (QC) procedures in the

---

(a) The following modification was voted on and added at the June 18-19, 2001, Steering Committee meeting at NRC Headquarters, Rockville, Maryland:

"Additional Federal organizations may become parties to this MOU by petitioning the Steering Committee and signing an Addendum to the MOU. The Addendum will commit the new Federal cooperating organization to assume the obligations and rights of MOU membership as specified in the established MOU, dated July 5, 2001. The parties to the MOU agree to delegate the authority to the Steering Committee to review requests for MOU membership and to approve additional parties. The Steering Committee Chair will sign the requester's Addendum to indicate approval of the agencies that are parties to this MOU."

development and use of these research and modeling products. Specific QA/QC issues will be resolved during the development of the specific IAG's.

h.   Effective date: This MOU will become effective upon the date of signature of the last cooperating Federal Agency to execute the MOU and will continue in force for 5 years or until modified or terminated by mutual consent.

Ashok Thadani, Director
Office of Nuclear Regulatory Research
U.S. Nuclear Regulatory Commission

Henry L. Longest II, Senior Resource Official
Office of Research and Development
U.S. Environmental Protection Agency

James R. Houston, PhD, Director
Engineer Research and Development Center
U.S. Army Corps of Engineers

Gerald G. Boyd, Deputy Assistant Secretary
Office of Science and Technology
U.S. Department of Energy

Robert M. Hirsch, PhD, Associate Director for Water
U.S. Geological Survey
Department of the Interior

Floyd P. Horn, PhD, Administrator
Agricultural Research Service
U.S. Department of Agriculture

NRC FORM 335
(2-89)
NRCM 1102,
3201, 3202

U.S. NUCLEAR REGULATORY COMMISSION

BIBLIOGRAPHIC DATA SHEET

(See instructions on the reverse)

1. REPORT NUMBER
(Assigned by NRC, Add Vol., Supp., Rev., and Addendum Numbers, if any.)

NUREG/CP-0177
PNNL-13654

2. TITLE AND SUBTITLE

Proceedings of the Enviromental Software Systems Compatibility and Linkage Workshop

Hosted by U.S. Nuclear Regulatory Commission, NRC Professional Development Center, Rockville, Maryland, March 7-9, 2000

3. DATE REPORT PUBLISHED

MONTH	YEAR
May	2002

4. FIN OR GRANT NUMBER

5. AUTHOR(S)

Gene Whelan, PNNL, and Thomas J. Nicholson, NRC

6. TYPE OF REPORT

Technical

7. PERIOD COVERED *(Inclusive Dates)*

March 7-9, 2000

8. PERFORMING ORGANIZATION - NAME AND ADDRESS *(If NRC, provide Division, Office or Region, U.S. Nuclear Regulatory Commission, and mailing address; if contractor, provide name and mailing address.)*

Pacific Northwest National Laboratory
P.O. Box 999
Richland, WA 99352

9. SPONSORING ORGANIZATION - NAME AND ADDRESS *(If NRC, type "Same as above"; if contractor, provide NRC Division, Office or Region, U.S. Nuclear Regulatory Commission, and mailing address.)*

Division of Systems Analysis and Regulatory Effectiveness
Office of Nuclear Regulatory Research
U.S. Nuclear Regulatory Commission
Washington, DC 20555-0001

10. SUPPLEMENTARY NOTES

Federal Interagency MOU on Multimedia Environmental Modeling

11. ABSTRACT *(200 words or less)*

The NRC hosted a Federal interagency workshop on multimedia environmental software systems and data systems. The "Environmental Software Systems Compatibility and Linkage Workshop" was held at NRC 's Professional Development Center in Rockville, MD, on March 7-9, 2000. The environmental software systems that were discussed are used to evaluate contaminant release, transport and health effects through various media (hence multimedia refers to air, ground, and surface water) and environmental pathways to the public. A major motivation for the workshop was the desire of the participating Federal agencies to realize efficiencies and cost savings by utilizing existing models, systems, and databases developed in their programs, rather than developing totally new systems. Workshop participants for this inaugural gathering included Federal agencies, their cooperators and contractors (e.g., U.S. Army Corps of Engineers, EPA's national exposure research laboratories, Offices of Research and Development, Radiation and Indoor Air, Solid Waste and Water, DOE, Pacific Northwest National Laboratory, Argonne National Laboratory, Golder Associates Inc., State of New Jersey and New Jersey Institute of Technology). The workshop objective was to facilitate communication between software products by focusing on standard attributes, protocols and specifications for linking environmental and risk models to databases and modeling systems. The workshop included presentations and demonstrations of current software systems (e.g., RESRAD, MEPAS, FRAMES, SEDSS, DandD, HWIR, LMS, WMS, etc.) used in site decommissioning assessments. The workshop attendees (1) reviewed detailed suggestions from system developers and users on attributes for linking the existing models, systems, Web-based, and GIS databases; and (2) discussed alternative software designs to ensure compatibility and linkage for future models, systems, and datasets. During an evening breakout session, the Federal agency

12. KEY WORDS/DESCRIPTORS *(List words or phrases that will assist researchers in locating the report.)*

decommissioning assessments
environmental database
environmental software systems
GIS-databases
MOU on Multimedia Enviromental models
risk assessment models
software design
software platform
software systems

13. AVAILABILITY STATEMENT

unlimited

14. SECURITY CLASSIFICATION

(This Page)

unclassified

(This Report)

unclassified

15. NUMBER OF PAGES

16. PRICE

NRC FORM 335 (2-89)

This form was electronically produced by Elite Federal Forms, Inc.

www.ingramcontent.com/pod-product-compliance
Lightning Source LLC
Chambersburg PA
CBHW080412290526
45791CB00008BA/2244